Yuichi Kawada is an experienced Shiatsu Master, heir to an old family tradition. A graduate of official schools and an early initiate, he has practiced and taught Shiatsu worldwide for many years.

Stephen Karcher, Ph.D, has worked with divinatory texts for more than thirty years as both scholar and consultant. He is generally acknowledged to be one of the world's experts on the psychological and spiritual uses of divination and the relation of divination to the arts. Among Karcher's publications are *The Kuan Yin Oracle* and *Symbols of Love*.

Also by Stephen Karcher

The Kuan Yin Oracle
Symbols of Love
Total I Ching

Essential Shiatsu

The Eight Extraordinary Meridians

Using the Japanese art of healing massage for
personal health and spiritual well-being

Yuichi Kawada
with Stephen Karcher

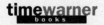

A *Time Warner* Book

First published in Great Britain in 2002
by Time Warner Books

Copyright © Yuichi Kawada and Stephen Karcher 2002

Illustrations by Dave Saunders

A CIP catalogue record for this book
is available from the British Library

ISBN 0 316 85949 4

Typeset in Cochin by M Rules
Printed and bound in Great Britain by
Clays Ltd, St Ives plc

Time Warner Books UK
Brettenham House
Lancaster Place
London WC2E 7EN

www.TimeWarnerBooks.co.uk

Contents

Preface

It is a great pleasure to write a few words on the occasion of the publication of Yuichi Kawada's book. I have known Yuichi Kawada for many years and I received Shiatsu treatment from him. I greatly respect his skill and his knowledge. I am, of course, not qualified to express an opinion about the mechanism that makes Shiatsu such an efficient method of making the mind and body work harmoniously. The importance of the psychosomatic aspect in the maintenance of our health is today well recognized by scientists coming from many different directions, but it seems we are only at the beginning of a deeper understanding. Yuichi Kawada's book will be very useful here, for it centres around a technique that is the outcome of a long period of personal experimentation. It may encourage people to use this method to help achieve a harmonious balance between body and mind and stimulate research on the neurophysiologic aspects that make Shiatsu effective.

Ilya Prigogine, Nobel Laureate

Foreword

This book is the product of much thought and practice. It is my sincere wish that what I have found over the years may be of help to you. The most fundamental ideas of Shiatsu, a discipline in which I have spent my entire life, are to serve and to help. It helps us restore the great natural balance of the individual and the world. Over many years I realized that we had need of something quite special to do this. The discovery of Essential Shiatsu and the Eight Extraordinary Meridians came out of my awareness of this need.

Essential Shiatsu or *Yoseido* combines the preventative care of traditional Shiatsu and its Twelve Principal Meridians with the crucial role of the Eight Extraordinary Meridians as rescue and emergency forces. It also draws on traditional eastern wisdom such as the *I Ching* and *The Yellow Emperor's Classic of Internal Medicine* to help us understand the interrelatedness of the world around us and the importance of the *Tao* or Way of Heaven and Earth. It is my experience that this combination of human love, philosophical insight and healing techniques can be of enormous benefit. I hope that you, too, might share this experience through the techniques presented in this book.

I am honoured to receive such warm, encouraging words from Dr Prigogine on the occasion of the publication of this book. I want to deeply and affectionately thank my wife Lydia, who supported me throughout its writing. I would also like to thank my very old friend Anne Colcord for her unflagging help and understanding, and Stephen Karcher for his editorial help and insight.

In the fullness of my heart, I offer this work to the spirit of my father, who taught me the way of Shiatsu when I was a very small boy.

Yuichi Kawada

Introduction

Shiatsu: The Art of the Open

Life is not a mystery, but an art
We have not fully uncarved.

Shiatsu is a contemporary bodywork therapy that operates on all the different energy levels of the body: physical, emotional/psychological and spiritual. The word 'shiatsu' literally means finger pressure (*shi*=fingers, *atsu*=pressure). The Japanese Ministry of Health and Welfare defines it as 'a form of manipulation administered by the thumbs, fingers and palms without the use of instruments . . . to apply pressure to the human skin in order to correct internal malfunction, promote and maintain health and treat specific diseases.'

Shiatsu seeks to heal people by joining forces with a person's natural healing ability. In particular it works with the adjustment and maintenance of the bone structure, joints, tendons, muscles and meridian lines or energy channels, whose malfunction distorts body energy and disrupts the functioning of the autonomous nervous system, thus causing disorder and disease.

Through touch it works directly with *ki* or *chi*, the 'basic psycho-physical spirit-energy' that links all other elements. This is the wonderful thing about Shiatsu.

In Japan, Shiatsu was recognized as a legitimate healing therapy about seventy-five years ago. Tokujiro Namikoshi initiated the first style of Shiatsu as we know it. He combined the diagnostic and treatment philosophy of acupuncture with the massage form known as *anma* to create a powerful healing art.

Oriental, specifically Chinese, medicine had developed a system of treating people by stimulating points on the skin that were connected to the functioning of internal organs. Imaginary lines that formed meridians, the channels through which energy (*ki* or *chi*) flows in the body, connected these points. The organs themselves were seen as much more than simply physiological. They were centres and 'orbits' of emotion, behaviour, association and inspiration as well as deep systemic functions. The 'organs' and their interconnections – all manifestations of the flow and coalescence of *ki*-energy – were the deep presence and function of a person's entire being. The discovery or re-discovery of the profound healing potential of traditional medicine was part of the great late nineteenth- and early twentieth-century re-imagining of traditional ways that occurred both east and west.

Shiatsu in Japan is different to Shiatsu in the west. Contemporary Japanese practice is very physical, involving deep tissue manipulation and aggressive stretches that westerners find difficult to accept. Also, the range of emotional expression in Japanese practice is severely restricted, reflecting the culture's deep social repression of feeling. Inspired by the contact of traditional teachers and new horizons however, there has been a great flowering of styles in the west: Barefoot Shiatsu, Macrobiotic Shiatsu, Namikoshi, Ohashiatsu, Shiatsu-Do, Zen Shiatsu, Healing-Shiatsu and Essential Shiatsu are great examples. They are all new, valid and very interesting ways of practising Shiatsu with different emphases on techniques and philosophy.

Shiatsu is not a clearly defined therapeutic technique in the western sense. Rather, the art or practice of Shiatsu is a continuum; a mixture of philosophy, self-help and professional expertise, exercises and stretches, thoughts on living, and a sophisticated system of intuitive diagnosis with an implicit spiritual background. It is communicated by experienced practitioners to be used by all. It is a way of life, a philosophy, an effective home remedy and a profound system of diagnosis and healing. This is a different kind of coherence than standard western models of therapeutic techniques. By diagnosing and responding to the phenomenon at hand on all levels and thus mobilizing the body-mind's innate healing power, Shiatsu breaks the contemporary categories of standard medicine both east and west.

For the centre of Shiatsu is not the intellectual systems and categories of diagnosis and evaluation, either 'diseases' or 'syndromes', usually seen in contemporary western medicine or post-revolution 'Traditional Chinese Medicine'. The centre of Shiatsu is a traditional 'woman's mystery' of touch, maternal affection, compassion and careful attention to what is there, to what 'presents itself'. In this sense it is a quite radical 'art of the open'.

Though thoroughly grounded in the basic techniques and discoveries of Chinese medicine and medical philosophy that entered Japan about a thousand years ago, the real ancestor of shiatsu is *anma*, a distinct form of healing and relaxing massage traditionally practiced by women and by the blind. *Anma* is very old, but it flourished particularly during the Edo period (about three hundred years ago) as a sophisticated method of diagnosis and treatment that included the Chinese herbal apothecary. It saw the body in terms of the flow of energy through the organs and meridians and sought to influence this energy through pressure at the *tsubo* or key 'pressure points'. *Anma* or *ankyo* (Chinese *amma*) and the exercises and stretches associated with it, called *do-in*, are discussed in *The Yellow Emperor's Classic of Internal Medicine* (Huangdi Neijing), a fundamental text in oriental medicine and philosophy that dates to about 400 BCE. They are mentioned there as particularly effective in dealing with the 'maladies of the centre'; physical and psychological disorders that afflict dwellers in the prosperous central plains where 'people enjoy eating without hard labour and a general weakness is prevalent'. Thus *ankyo* and *do-in*, in the new form of *shiatsu*, were considered very effective methods to deal with our own industrialized and post-industrialized 'affluent societies'.

There is a particular sense of time and origin central to these healing methods which we might call a 'golden age' that still exists as an innate healing potential within the body. So the emphasis in Shiatsu on treating 'what presents itself' is not really to cure a specific disease. It seeks to mobilize the body's innate health and healing capacity, leading it back through a series of 'karmic' causes and effects to a sense of that original power and purity. In this perspective, people's troubles become a part of their healing rather than something to simply be overcome in order to get better.

The core of this is 'being in touch'. Shiatsu practitioners often speak of themselves as 'manual workers'. A Shiatsu proverb states: 'Real medicine begins when the doctor puts her hands on the patient's *hara*,' which is the key abdominal area and a source that displays all that happens in the body. Shiatsu requires that the therapist directly experience the client's *ki* from the *hara*, which involves suspending the intellectual process until after the diagnosis has been made and the relevant meridians explored.

This diagnostic process, called *setsu-shin*, takes precedence over analytical or abstract considerations. Direct contact with the other, and the intuition that proceeds from that contact, is primary. And at the centre of *setsu-shin* is compassion and care towards the individual. Touching diagnosis is 'maternal affection towards the patient to feel her or his pain. We are not treating a problem, we are sharing the pain.' Though backed up by a sophisticated treatment cosmology based on yin–yang and five-process (*wuxing*) thinking, plus a wide vocabulary of 'skilful means' or treatment styles, this basic process focuses on something like the west's sense of 'healing hands', or the healing touch of a king or sage. It affirms the power of human contact, the touch communication between practitioner and patient, and a personal and 'holistic' sense of health and healing almost completely lacking in modern western medicine.

This sensitive 'feeling-with' is what you can and should expect from a Shiatsu practitioner, as well as specific tactical advice on changes that can help resolve your situation. It is a treatment that moves toward allowing the hidden causes of your complaint to manifest. Shiatsu relies on and seeks to further the healing capacity of good human relationships, an understanding through touch and body pressure, as well as mobilizing natural self-healing powers.

Shiatsu treatments usually extend over a period of time, with each session dealing with what 'presents itself' in the moment. You can expect an immediate sense of relaxation and relief, often coupled later with a temporary intensification of symptoms as your body's re-activated healing power discharges them. This is directly conveyed through the practitioner's touch: a firm, steady pressure on key points that relax the sympathetic nervous system and allow the body to adjust the function of the internal organs.

This openness and focus on the individual is one reason that westerners are now seeking out Shiatsu and related healing arts. People are becoming profoundly disillusioned by western allopathic medicine's impersonal perspective, the horrendous side-effects of some of its 'cures', and its complete non-recognition of a whole range of problems. These problems, which are one of Shiatsu's main concerns, can be summarized in a very well-known phrase: 'Disease is an indication we are not living properly'. Shiatsu seeks to give back to the individual the power over their own health. Though it offers treatments for specific disorders, Shiatsu does not look for disease as such but at the 'unhealthy phenomenon occurring in a specific individual'. Treatment is selected according to the specific phenomenon observed, not the treatment of a general disease syndrome.

Thus Shiatsu is preventative in the best sense. It treats the phenomenon before it develops into a specific disease, using not only finger-pressure techniques but also exercises, lifestyle changes and 'healthy ideas' about living in this world that can be incorporated into daily life. It sensitizes people to their own physical make-up so that they know immediately when something is 'not right'. The majority of people treated in a Shiatsu practice are what might be called 'half-healthy' or 'next-to-sick'. (In Japan, treatments are regularly provided free of charge to workers.) Western medicine really has no way to help these people until they become truly 'ill' in a recognized medical sense, that is until they develop a recognized disease or injury that requires major intervention. Studies show that most of those who come to and are significantly helped by a Shiatsu practitioner are suffering from muscular-skeletal disorders, psychological stress or depression, digestive complaints such as irritable bowel syndrome, neurological complaints such as migraine or hypertension, or need help in dealing with side-effects of chemical treatments for cancer or HIV.

Diagnosis in Shiatsu reflects how the body and the mind are responding to stimuli and focuses on their ability to adapt to changing circumstances. 'Being in touch' (*setsu-shin*) on any level of practice is simultaneously providing acquaintance, observation and treatment. It will not only deliver objective information about the person being treated, it will open a space between practitioner and patient through the embodied mind. It creates the room to experience, enabling the patient to become aware of the nature and origin of her or his own disturbance.

In our society, many people are searching for a new sense of meaning in their life and the ability to take responsibility for their own health. Ideas found in acupuncture and Shiatsu, in which a physical approach and a deep sense of spirituality go hand in hand, and in which the patient has the central role, have a positive attraction in the evolving alternative movements in western society. Shiatsu is directly linked with Japanese martial arts such as Aikido and its practice is often described in terms of the revelation of the flow of energy in quantum physics or in Buddhist meditation. Its diagnosis is not looking to see something, but waiting for something to be shown.

Shiatsu is about making connections; connections to heaven that waken and brighten us, helping us to reach health, happiness and peace, and connections to earth that let us fulfill the purpose of our lives, to bring our spiritual potential into the 'real life'. The actual practice of Shiatsu, through its connecting of heaven and earth, its heart-to-heart contact and its sense of 'being in touch' outside of space and time, is a spiritual experience. It can help to give someone a taste of their spiritual potential and fragrance, a benefit to every aspect of their life.

This is the context in which Yuichi Kawada developed *Yoseido* or Essential Shiatsu, with its unique emphasis on the healing power of the Eight Extraordinary Meridians, a great aid in our 'troubled times'. In this book we see his mind and his practice at work in a range of specific techniques for both practitioner and lay person, exercises and stretches, 'aids to right living', and some ground-breaking theoretical observations connected with that fundamental Eastern classic *I Ching* or *Classic of Change*. I could do no better than to let him introduce the inspiration and concern that gave birth to *Yoseido* and the Eight Extraordinary Meridians.

Our world is filled with unresolved problems. From cancer and AIDS to social upheavals, society is riddled with crises of identity. New religious sects appear, prophesying paradise and victimizing those who seek answers in the midst of confusion. The family has broken down. There is no moral authority. Crime is an everyday affair. We no longer 'belong' in the world.

In a small way, Essential Shiatsu and my work with the Eight Extraordinary Meridians is a step towards bringing back a sense of belonging. The promise of a perfect world that is found in the Bible and other great scriptures is not merely a utopian dream to happen at the end of the world.

Our inner selves are bound up with our outer bodies. Each part helps the other and they follow along the desirable path. When you burn your hand, your whole body hurts. Consider the way we walk. When one leg moves, the other stops and stays in place. This frees the first leg. When it reaches its destination, it supports the other, freeing it in its turn. This is harmonious progression. It is how we walk on the Way.

For me, this book and the work it represents form a small contribution towards bringing people together and enhancing their sense of belonging to one another. This circle extends to families, friends and acquaintances, radiating ever outward. *Essential Shiatsu* is, I feel, a means of helping people realize within themselves the purpose of existence. This practice can return us to a state of belonging as one big family. Heaven, earth and humans must move forward together if we are to understand the purpose and meaning of life on this planet.

Shiatsu is now being used in a wide range of contexts, therapies and movement arts. There are recognized Shiatsu organizations in most western countries that will be happy to give you information about practitioners, programmes and how to become a Shiatsu practitioner yourself. You can contact Yuichi Kawada through his website at http://www.shiatsu-yoseido.com. Here are a few books you might find interesting:

Bonnie Bainbridge Cohen: *Sensing, Thinking and Feeling*
A classic of bodywork and its relation to the healing and movement arts.

Peter den Dekker: 'In Search of Style: The Role of TCM in Shiatsu Practice' in *Journal of Shiatsu and Oriental Body Therapy*
A fascinating consideration of the 'open' nature of diagnosis in Shiatsu contrasted with the contemporary development of 'Traditional Chinese Medicine' in the People's Republic.

Shudo Denmei: *Meridian Therapy* (Eastland Press, 1990)
A modern classic on the contemporary eastern theory of therapy through work on the energy meridians.

David G. Jamison: *Shiatsu and Orthodox Medicine*
This examines the ways in which oriental medicine is viewed by established western practice.

Stanley Keleman: *Emotional Anatomy* (Center Press, 1985)
Not Shiatsu related, but gives a great sense of body configurations and processes in imagining the emotions.

Elaine Liechti: *The Complete Illustrated Guide to Shiatsu* (Element, 1999)

Carola Beresford–Cooke: *Shiatsu Theory and Practice* (Churchill Livingstone, 1995)
Two good overall presentations of the field, with history, theory and practical examples.

Giovanni Macciocia: *The Foundations of Chinese Medicine* (Churchill Livingstone, 1989)

> Perhaps the best contemporary textbook on traditional Chinese medicine, with a chapter on the Eight Extraordinary Meridians and their basic functions.

Shizuto Masunaga: *Zen Shiatsu* and *Zen Imagery Exercises* (Japan Publications (USA), 1997)

> Radical and exciting revisions of Shiatsu by one of the greatest of its practitioners and theorists.

Mark Seem: *A New American Acupuncture* (Blue Poppy Press, 2000)

> A contemporary practitioner describes how he uses the Eight Extraordinary Meridians in all kinds of pain treatments.

1

The Way of Care

Essential Shiatsu presents a combination of the care inherent in Shiatsu, the philosophy or wisdom of the *I Ching* or *Classic of Change*, and my very new discovery of how we can use the Eight Extraordinary Meridians to heal the great imbalances that afflict us as inhabitants of an industrialized and polluted world.

The first thing we must understand in order to see into this combination of things is the notion of *ki* or energy. This *ki*, shown in the Chinese character as 'steam cooking rice', represents an energy force present in all things. Everything has *ki*. In its refined form *ki* moves and flows almost invisibly, like steam. In its denser aspects it coalesces into bodies, like rice. Thus everything is living and interconnected.

In oriental medicine, *ki* energy is thought of in terms of yin and yang. The word yin shows us something enclosed, the shadowed side of a hill that is not exposed to the sun. It is something that is hidden inside. The word yang, on the contrary, shows us the sun shining brightly, rising above a hill. All is exposed to the light; nothing is hidden.

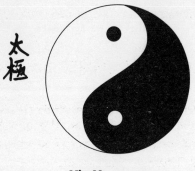

Yin Yang

Everything is constantly moving and changing between these two complementary principles. They do not exist separately, for each contains the seed of the other. According to Taoist thought, these two forces were born out of the primal chaos, and when they separated and stabilized our world came into being. The balance between them is what maintains our existence. Oriental medicine as a whole is primarily concerned with correcting an imbalance between these two forces. This imbalance is the basic cause of sickness and destructive energy.

It is important to note that yin and yang are not rigid definitions. In Shiatsu they represent a dynamic system of describing the condition of a person at a given moment, in a given situation. Thus feet can be 'yin' – that is, stabilizing and structuring – in context of their place in the body order yet, in terms of motion and action, can also function as 'yang', that is, initiating movement and being instrumental in changing positions. A good practitioner of oriental medicine is constantly shifting these categories.

SHIATSU AND INNER BALANCE

Shiatsu is a form of therapy that works directly on the body. It involves direct contact, the manipulation of specific points on the body, and a series of stretches and exercises. Shiatsu manipulation uses the thumbs and the palms of the hands to put pressure on a particular *meridian*, or energy-circulating channel. By doing this, we can adjust the balance of yin and yang within an individual. We can liberate tension and redirect blocked energy. This promotes a free flow of *ki* energy and makes you aware of the energy connections between your body and the rest of the world. In order to do this, the Shiatsu practitioner, whether lay person or professional, must be in good order, with correct posture and proper breathing. Most of all, when practising Shiatsu we must relax and concentrate on our own state of mind. If we are clear of negative thinking – anger, worry, sadness – and focus on the points we are pressing, then the breathing and the flow come naturally.

Essential Shiatsu is based on the flow of *ki* energy through the body as a reflection of the interconnection of heaven and earth. According to oriental medicine,

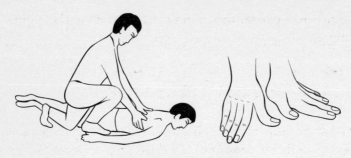

Practitioner at work

our bodies channel energy through Twelve Principal Meridians and Eight Extraordinary Meridians.

The meridians are arranged in pairs: one is a yang meridian that handles communication and interchange, while the other is a yin meridian that acts as a reservoir of energy. Energy circulates through these meridians each day, to nourish them and to deploy defensive energies to deal with changes in weather, diet, physical movement or psychological stress.

Because our bodies are constantly harassed by imbalance, the Eight Extraordinary Meridians have the purpose of controlling imbalanced energy in the Twelve Principal Meridians. A fundamental text of Chinese medicine, the *Nangio*, discusses one of their main functions as the absorption of excess energy from the Principal Meridians, which are then left free to equalize the normal bodily flow. The Extraordinary Meridians thus can be seen as canals or dykes, created to relieve an overflow of energy in an emergency. They are vital to understanding the dynamics of energy moving in the body. Many meditation techniques focus on these

meridians in order to attain both longevity and enlightenment.

LIVING IN THE WORLD

For thousands of years different ways of caring for the
body, such as acupuncture, have been practised in
China. By the sixth century the Chinese had developed
specific techniques to help people living in the great
cities, and these procedures were imported into Japan
and developed over many years. Shiatsu grew out of
combining old Japanese healing methods such as *ankyo*
and *∂o-in*, which stimulated energy flow in the meridians, with these Chinese forms of acupuncture and
herbal medicine. It was reinvented or rediscovered in
the 1920s and recognized by the Japanese government
as an official form of medicine.

Shiatsu is primarily a way to understand and live
with the interconnections between heaven and earth as
they are manifested in your own body. It can help
people suffering from specific complaints, but it was
not designed for that. In Japan, you do not use Shiatsu
when you are sick; you use it to stay in good health. If
you come to me with a stomach disorder, I can treat it,
but ideally it never should have gone that far. We
should have seen the disequilibrium, the imbalanced
energy, and worked on the points necessary to eliminate
the problem before it happened.

Today our relationship to what eastern thought calls
heaven and earth seems quite disharmonious. We live in

an age of ecological disasters – global warming, over-population, deforestation and acid rain, degradation of the ozone layer, pollution – that show a profound imbalance between heaven and earth. This imbalance is directly caused by human beings. If we are to live harmoniously with heaven and earth and the constant energy flow that occurs between them, we must develop personal insight and an understanding of this delicate balance. Shiatsu helps us experience this intricate harmony and find a way to successfully participate in it.

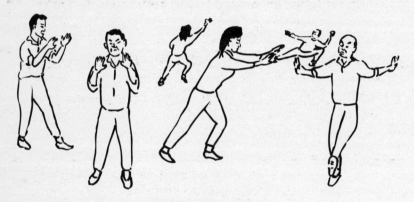

Performing t'ai chi

A basic tenet of oriental medicine is that what occurs within the body is directly connected to the movements of heaven and earth, sky, land and sea. Ancient people thought that a long, healthy life was a direct consequence of respecting the movements of heaven and earth. Heaven gives us the four seasons and the four stages of transformation: birth (*sei*) and spring; growing (*chiyo*) and summer; harvest (*shiyu*) and autumn; and stocking up (*zo*) and winter. They felt that to stay healthy you must attune yourself to the cyclic flow of these natural forces and adjust your activities to them. Movements in our body mirror the movements of heaven and earth and stem from their interaction. If your body is sick, you have somehow abused heaven and earth's energies.

From this perspective, heaven and earth have regular cycles. The energy of heaven is expressed as wind, heat, humidity, dryness and cold. These elements descend from the atmosphere and combine with earth energy to produce the tastes – acid, bitter, sweet, spicy, salty – which have a direct effect on human organs. *The Yellow Emperor's Classic of Internal Medicine* states that energy flow in the body is deeply affected by the interaction of heaven and earth. To find a balance within ourselves, the energy of the body, which moves through the meridians, must flow freely. Such a free flow of personal *ki* is achieved through diet, breathing, exercise and manipulation. The transformation of the seasons also changes the forms of the plants around us, the main source of what we eat and drink, so our food, too, should follow the change of the seasons. Therefore, wherever possible, eat food that is available in the season in which it naturally grows and, ideally, has been grown in the area in which you live. Thus you will be more in tune with the natural rhythms and this automatically has a positive effect on the body. There are, of course, staple foods such as rice and grains but one eats, for example, squashes and root vegetables in autumn and winter, fresh greens in spring, and fruits as they naturally ripen. A good book on this is *Recipes for Self-Healing* by David Leggett (Totnes: Merdian Press, 1999) which gives a range of recipes and food choices based on principles of Chinese medicine.

THE PRACTICE OF SHIATSU

Shiatsu is not simply a therapeutic technique in the western sense. Rather, the art or practice of Shiatsu is a mixture of philosophy, self-help, exercises and stretches, thoughts on living, massage techniques and sophisticated diagnosis. It is a way of life, a philosophy, an effective home remedy and an expert system of diagnosis and healing. It is taught by experienced practitioners to be used by all.

To practise Shiatsu, to use the techniques as a therapist or an amateur, we need discipline. To learn Shiatsu, we need form. Life itself has a natural form: breathing. Humans and animals in particular must breathe to live, and our lives are controlled and characterized by breathing. Form is important to the practice of Shiatsu, for we work with regular patterns and orderly sequences of pressure points.

It is also of crucial importance that we do not fall into the rigid form of mechanical repetition. Form is important, but what is essential exists beyond the form. The essence of movement is breathing. And, in turn, smooth, calm breathing is dependent upon a composed state of mind. Your state of mind regulates your breathing and your posture, not the other way around. This is why *The Yellow Emperor's Classic of Internal Medicine* emphasized the supreme importance of mastering the emotions of greed, desire, passion, sadness and obsession.

FEELING CONNECTED

So, first of all, doing Shiatsu requires a disciplined and composed state of mind. Without this, we cannot deliver healing energy to the person we are working on. In Japan, many blind people work as masseurs (*amma*). They have a much more subtle and effective sense of touch than sighted people do. Because they cannot see the outside world of images and desires, they are able to concentrate everything within. This inner darkness brings a special atmosphere of calmness and uniformity, a deep feeling of connection or oneness with others.

Shiatsu practitioners have to create a special atmosphere to experience this sense of being connected or being one with our patients. There are several ways to do this. Daily breathing and meditation exercises concentrate the feeling of connection. Doing the Extraordinary Meridian Stretching Exercises each day is another effective method. When the energy circulates in the right way our mind naturally becomes attuned to the feeling of oneness. In a larger sense this indicates that we are connecting the energies of heaven and earth. The more we can free ourselves of obsessions and compulsive ideas, the more the energy of heaven and earth flows into us. In this sense the Shiatsu treatment is no longer in our hands, but in the control of the infinitely abundant energies of heaven and earth.

In oriental philosophy we must first find a harmony in the self before we can join with the universal forces. If the *ki* is flowing freely within us, harmony with the universal forces will occur almost automatically. In Taoist terms, the way of individual harmony leads on to the Way of Heaven. This process of exchanging energy is circular and infinite.

THE PROPER WAY TO LIVE

The Yellow Emperor's Classic of Internal Medicine gives us an important insight into regulating our lives. There are several versions of this book; I rely on the Japanese translation by Yojozen. The *I Ching* or *Classic of Change* is often mentioned in this book too, as is the name of the founder of Taoism, Lao-tzü. It is strongly coloured with Taoist philosophy.

To explain the workings of the meridians the Yellow Emperor uses the officials of a national government as an analogy. The Spleen-Pancreas meridian can be seen as the body's finance minister, the Kidney meridian as the defence minister, and the Liver meridian as the commander-in-chief of the army. The prime minister, the Lung meridian, is in charge of the government, and the emperor, the Heart meridian, is the symbol of the nation, the unifier of national identity. The prime minister and the emperor work together each day to keep the nation functioning smoothly.

Physiologically, the Heart and Lung meridians also work together. The Heart meridian is linked with the blood, and the Lung meridian is linked with *ki*, or subtle energy. In oriental medicine *ki* and blood are inseparable. As long as there is life, *ki* is present in the blood, guiding it and enhancing its quality.

According to this old text, the key to a long, healthy life is harmonizing (*chiyo*) the divine force or *shin* that dwells in the Heart meridian. We may do this through harmonizing breath and posture (*kei*) and by unifying the psychic entities associated with each organ: Liver (*kon*), Lungs (*haku*), Kidneys (*sei*) and Spleen-Pancreas (*I*). The spirit *kon* in the Liver is particularly linked with *shin*, divine force, while the spirit *haku* in the Lungs is particularly linked with *sei*, breathing and posture. *Shin* or divine force co-ordinates all psychological manifestations of human behaviour.

To live harmoniously means to follow the movement of nature and the interaction of heaven and earth as fully as possible, while keeping your *shin* intact. To do this you must curb excessive desire, greed and obsession with things. The ancient Chinese suggested that we could do this by always putting ourselves below the power of heaven, and were very sceptical of people who tried to appropriate it. If the emperor, through his egotism, forgot the power of heaven the people would revolt and establish a new emperor who would listen to heaven's command rather than his own will.

Lao-tzü said that to return to the source of things in nature is to find your own deep happiness. Our role is to follow the constantly interacting forces of heaven and earth and thus become an integral part of the natural design of the cosmos. This is one of my own deepest convictions, something I seek to promote in all the work that I do.

2

The Elements of Essential Shiatsu

I conceived the idea of Essential Shiatsu or *Yoseido* as a way to deal with imbalances in our bodies by working directly on the Extraordinary Meridians, the emergency channels of the body's energy flow. *Yoseido* or Essential Shiatsu emphasizes the importance of understanding and using the Eight Extraordinary Meridians through exercise and stretching, learning and using the regulatory and diagnostic points. It integrates this use with the basic knowledge of Shiatsu on posture, breathing, attitude of the practitioner and the central importance of oriental philosophy and the *I Ching* or *Classic of Change*. *Yoseido* is based on the idea of nourishing your life force by freely circulating the energy of heaven and earth within your body. *Yo* means to nourish; *Sei* refers to your physical life force; *Do* refers to the Way, the way we understand and experience this energy; *Yoseido* means harmonizing your individual life energy by experiencing the interaction of the energies of heaven and earth.

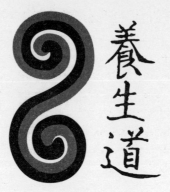

Yoseido

The symbol for Essential Shiatsu or *Yoseido* exemplifies this interaction. The upper part of the symbol refers to the action of heaven. It brings yang energy to the centre while showing there is a contrary interior yin movement that balances it. When yang is fully concentrated, it gives birth to yin. In the same way, the lower part of the symbol shows yin energy concentrating towards the centre. When it attains its maximum force it creates yang, which counterbalances the yin.

Yang dominates in heaven; it creates wind, heat, humidity, dryness and cold. It contains within itself the potential of yin. Yin dominates on earth, and gives birth to the five elements, wood, fire, earth, metal and water. It contains within itself the potential of yang.

THE CHARACTERS OF YIN AND YANG

Yin and yang are the basis of our constitution and affect everything we do in a treatment. But yin and yang are not the same in each of us. It is very important to distinguish the differences and to sense the different types of character and constitution involved. If you look at the illustrations, you can see the basic type of the yin and yang constitutions.

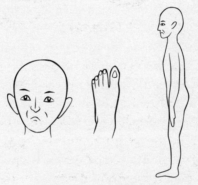

Yin-type constitution

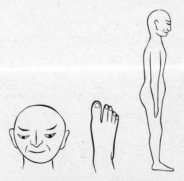

Yang-type constitution

The yin person has a triangular face and a small nose, large open eyes, small eyebrows and pointy, mouselike ears. The yang person, on the contrary, has a large nose, slanting eyes, large ears and large eyebrows. Seen from the side, the yang person will have a bulging abdomen. The feet show a distinct difference: the yin person has a pointed big toe, while the yang person has a rounded big toe.

In Shiatsu, the feet and toes are important diagnostic tools, for they are thought to have direct connection to internal organs. Many chronic problems show up on the toes. The yin person, for example, will often have very sharp toes, ears, nose and jaw, indicating overstimulation of the sympathetic nervous system.

Wide-open eyes show the development of the analytical brain, and are a symptom of our times. We need more and more conscious analytical skills to deal with technological advances and information overload. Because of the Internet, for example, we can reach around the globe with our fingers, without the need to travel. We sit in front of a screen, push on a keyboard and use those wide-open eyes, but the complete lack of leg exercise weakens our internal organs and leaves us open to all sorts of pollution, literal and spiritual. It destroys our body's defences. *The Yellow Emperor's Classic of Internal Medicine* diagnosed this condition 2,000 years ago: people who live in cities suffer from a lack of physical exercise. Several forms of healing arts, such as *do-in* and *ankyo*, were developed to deal with this problem. The Extraordinary Meridian Stretching Exercises serve the same purpose if you do them yourself each day.

We can add the system of the Five Processes to this

yin and yang typology to make it even more interesting. The Five Processes – wood, fire, earth, metal and water – are an old Chinese system of describing the character of things and the way that they change. The second group of illustrations shows the morphology of the faces of each of the Five Processes' characters. Each indicates certain characteristic weaknesses of the body, and this is the reason they are useful to us as healers. These faces typify ancient Chinese warriors.

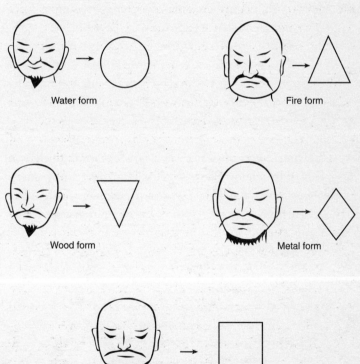

Water form

Fire form

Wood form

Metal form

Earth form

Five Process Types

- The **water process** face shows someone who is patient and understanding, with a real understanding of the other person's point of view. He is often a peacemaker. His weakness is in the Kidneys.

- The **fire process** face shows the superb mounted warrior, passionate, fearless and unpredictable. Unafraid of death, he will charge into the lion's mouth. He has little patience and is quite aggressive. The weakness of fire types is the Heart.

- The **wood process** type is an excellent tactician, a commander-in-chief. He is restrained, even cold-blooded, like Wellington confronting Napoleon at Waterloo. His weakness is the Liver.

- The **metal process** type is a professional soldier, a killer. He understands combat and has impressive endurance. His behaviour is predictable and he is an exemplary bodyguard. There are many of these metal types in professional sports today. His weakness is the Lungs.

- The **earth process** type is a good support soldier and can always be depended on. He helps keep up camp morale. He loves eating, drinking and sex, and fights not for the love of it, like the metal type, but out of necessity. His weakness is the Spleen and Pancreas.

It is important to remember that these faces are the result of habitual states of mind. If the state of mind changes, the form of the face will change accordingly, as will the ears, fingers and toes. The outer forms of things are directly connected with the state of our mind and our internal organs, which have an intelligence of their own. Over time, your state of mind can profoundly change your appearance.

THE TWELVE PRINCIPAL MERIDIANS

The Twelve Principal Meridians in our body move energy through the organs along the course shown in the Essential Shiatsu symbol. The Lung meridian, for example, which is paired with the Large Intestine meridian, is a yin meridian and moves out from the centre of the body. The Large Intestine meridian, its complement, is a yang meridian that moves from the extremities of the body, the fingertips, towards the centre of the body and the face. These represent the working of heaven. The Stomach meridian and the Spleen-Pancreas meridian together represent earth energy. The Stomach meridian is yang and moves from the centre towards the extremities, the feet. The Spleen-Pancreas meridian is a yin meridian, moving inwards from the feet towards the centre of the chest. The eight other Principal Meridians follow the same pattern. The model of this pattern is the symbol of Essential Shiatsu.

The idea of the internal body organs in Shiatsu is different than western medicine. Though they include the physical organs – Lung, Heart, Stomach and Spleen, Pancreas, Large and Small Intestine – these organs are thought of as centres of a series of functions, processes, emotions and styles of experience. For example, the Kidneys conserve life and push the organism to actualize its potential. They are the site of the essence (*jing*) or individual fate and transform the essence into available energy, controlling the flow of courage and fear. The Heart is master of the organs and home of the spirits that bring inspiration and joy. It commands the pathways and the blood, brings the spark of life and offers a quiet centre in which the spirits find a voice. The Spleen and Stomach stabilize and transform nourishment. They rot and ripen food, govern the free flow of ideas, control and protect central energy. The Liver rules the free flow of energy and emotion. It stimulates everything that moves or moves in the body, purifies the blood, links eyes and sexual organs, desire and anger, vision and motivation, giving the capacity to act decisively. The Lungs are connected with the skin and nervous system, regulating the rhythm of life, making energy descend and dispersing it throughout the body. They connect the surface with the central nervous system, and are involved in sexual stimulation and the power of inner images.

Meridians are named for and interconnect these organs and the fields of activity they represent. It is through the meridians and the points (*tsubo*) that we can influence the behaviour of the organs.

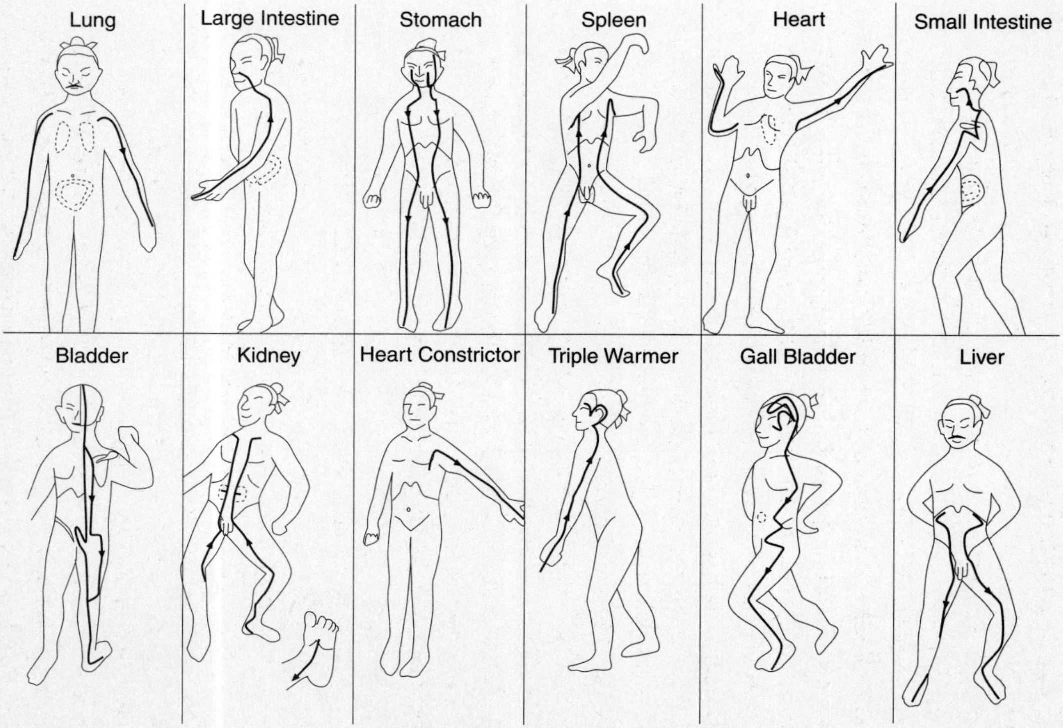

Small Intestine

Heart

Spleen

Stomach

Large Intestine

Lung

Liver

Gall Bladder

Triple Warmer

Heart Constrictor

Kidney

Bladder

Principal Meridians

```
┌─────────────────────────────────────────┐
│        12 Principle Meridians            │
│                  +                       │
│        5 Organs and 6 Inner Organs       │
└─────────────────────────────────────────┘
```

┌ Lung meridian (yin)
│ Large Intestine meridian (yang)
│ Stomach meridian (yang)
│ Spleen-Pancreas meridian (yin)
12 Principal │ Heart meridian (yin)
Meridians │ Small Intestine meridian (yang)
│ Bladder meridian (yang)
│ Kidney meridian (yin)
│ Heart Constrictor meridian (yin)
│ Triple Warmer meridian (yang)
│ Gall Bladder meridian (yang)
└ Liver meridian (yin)

┌ Lung
│ Spleen / Pancreas
5 Organs │ Heart
│ Kidney
└ Liver

┌ Large Intestine
│ Stomach
6 Inner │ Small Intestine
Organs │ Bladder
│ Triple Warmer
└ Gall Bladder

Principal Meridian Table

Each of the meridians connects a series of points, all of which have names and qualities in the traditional method of Shiatsu. Called 'dragon holes' by the Chinese, these are the places where we can apply pressure and affect the flow of energy. They are also places where one meridian connects with or 'crosses' another. You can learn the position of these points from a book like this one, then stimulate the points along a given meridian that feel blocked or enervated. You will recognize this by the tenderness, congestion, swelling or feeling of cold or emptiness when you touch the point. A firm, steady, responsive pressure for brief periods (10–30 seconds) is very helpful. In combination with a basic sense of which meridians affect a given problem, this can produce quite effective results. We all have the ability to recognize profoundly disturbed energy through the sense of touch, and the sense of care itself is, truly, a very healing thing. If you really want to learn the healing touch, however, I would very strongly recommend that you work with a practising Shiatsu Master. There are certain things that can only be taught in person, through direct transmission.

BREATHING TO CONNECT
HEAVEN AND EARTH

The most important aspect of the interchange between heaven and earth is breathing. Our breath is life itself; without it we cannot live more than a few minutes. We breathe constantly, and it is this process that permits energy to circulate through the meridians in our bodies.

Breathing involves four different meridians. When we breathe out, the Lung meridian and the Stomach meridian are very active, while the Large Intestine and Spleen-Pancreas meridians support the movement. When we breathe in the Large Intestine meridian and the Spleen-Pancreas meridian become very active while the Lung and Stomach meridians support their movement. When we exhale, the Lung and Stomach meridians are moving energy from the centre to the extremities of our bodies, whereas when we inhale the Large Intestine and Spleen-Pancreas meridians are moving energy towards the centre of our bodies. The Large Intestine and Spleen-Pancreas meridians move earth energy from the feet to the hands, while the Lung and Stomach meridians move heaven energy from the hands to the feet via the head.

If our breathing is shallow, laboured or weak, we slow the flow of these energies. Most breathing practices emphasize the importance of breathing out. This has a symbolic meaning. Exhalation is an emptying out of the self, letting go preconceived ideas of the world. Unless we can get rid of what we have collected and make space inside ourselves, we cannot replenish our bodies.

This is why so many breathing techniques concentrate on breathing out. Most healthy people have a longer exhalation period. Breathing out activates the Lung and Heart meridians, the two most important meridians in our body. An image for this breathing practice is the Zen Master who sits and meditates, breathing calmly, with long exhalations and a slow, calm heartbeat.

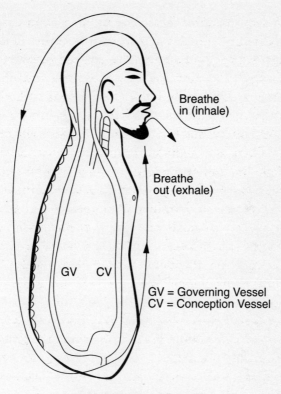

Breathe
in (inhale)

Breathe
out (exhale)

GV   CV

GV = Governing Vessel
CV = Conception Vessel

Yin and Yang Breathing

EXERCISES FOR KEEPING FIT EVERY DAY

Shiatsu is not just a matter of pressing the meridian points. Stretching and sitting postures play a key role in creating the basis for healing.

The following series of simple exercises can help to keep you healthy and open the way for deeper work.

They are best performed in the Japanese sitting position seen in the diagrams. Sitting in a chair will do, so long as the back is straight and your feet are parallel to the floor.

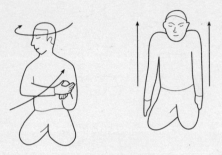

Simple stretch 1

Push one hand against the other wrist until you feel tension in your shoulder. At the same time, move your head in the opposite direction. As you do this, inhale. Exhale and repeat. Do this ten times on each side.

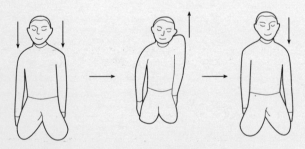

Simple stretch 2

Inhale and lift both shoulders. When you can no longer hold your breath, exhale suddenly and drop both shoulders. Repeat ten times with both shoulders, then ten times on each side.

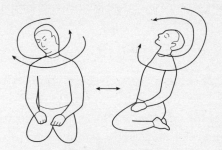

Simple stretch 3

Draw a large circle with the top of your head, both front and back. If your neck is supple, you are probably healthy; if it is stiff, there is probably a block or disorder somewhere in your body.

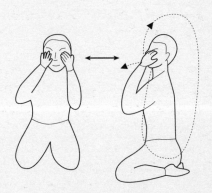

Simple stretch 4

Gently cover your eyes with your fingertips. Breathe in slowly. Close your eyes. Imagine you are taking the

energy of heaven down the back of your body through
the Governing Vessel to your coccyx. As you breathe
out, imagine you are bringing the energy back up the
front of your body through the Conception Vessel.
Repeat this twenty times.

These exercises are an extremely effective way to
cleanse the body of toxins and regenerate energy. They
offer a basis for healing and act as a preparation for the
stretching exercises directly connected with the Eight
Extraordinary Meridians and dealing with specific disorders and imbalances.

PREVENTING DISORDER

The Yellow Emperor's Classic of Internal Medicine, the *I
Ching* and oriental medicine in general are all concerned
with preventing disorder before it manifests itself. They
emphasize prevention as the highest form of the healing
arts. Prevention turns away negative energy before it
can take hold and overwhelm us.

Today our moral and spiritual values are being dis-
placed by empty rhetoric. Our loyalties and allegiances
are unstable and unreliable, and our ambition is disconnected from what is truly important in life. Despair,
destruction, depression and disaster are common. Sex,
violence, drugs and other short-term stimulants
abound. Humour and a sense of lightness are vanishing.
The desire for wholeness, a basic spiritual need, is
masked by short-term desires that feed a fantasy world

where the ideal is to feel good at any cost. This fantasy world takes the place of the real world that draws on our imagination, reason and the depths of our faculties and resources.

In the western tradition Christ showed us through the crucifixion that our body and our soul are united and that it is the soul that needs our attention. The need to find inner truth and contentment is a unifying thread, coupled with the injunction to 'love thy neighbour'. We must learn to belong, to join self-respect with respect for others. This is extremely important today. Sin and illness have parallel implications. We usually try to avoid pain and physical suffering. Like sin, we try to put sickness out of our mind, but it is only through sickness that we can understand what it means to be whole, just as it is only through sin that we can achieve redemption. When we abuse our bodies we become ill, and this suffering forces us to think about our actions, helping us rise to a better, more integrated state of being. Sin, too, offers us an opportunity to become aware of the world around us. Once confronted, it heightens our sense of belonging to a whole. The essential message is that we must keep firm contact with the earth while elevating our thoughts to heaven.

Traditional oriental medicine is preventative because its main aim is not just to eradicate the symptoms of sickness but to preserve and protect health. When sickness occurs, we consider how it may have started and how we can keep it from happening again. The symptom is always a lesson in the relation between harmony and disharmony.

The disharmony of sickness can force a person to become conscious of his actions. It can make someone learn the deep meaning of universal law as a perpetual flow, a sense of equilibrium. Modern medicine tends to make a diagnosis by analysing the nature of symptoms and deducing the cause of the illness. This approach neglects the body as an integrated whole as it ignores what the psychological state of the individual has contributed to the problem. Seeking the cause is not wrong, but it is only part of the answer. It is important to take a more inclusive, global view. Looking at the flow of yin and yang energies is the oriental way of arriving at a fuller picture of the body's difficulties, and it lets us include many things modern medicine has a tendency to overlook.

IMBALANCED ENERGY IN THE BODY

Imbalanced energy is directly manifested in the meridians, which influence the entire being. The energy imbalance in a specific point or area is either empty (*kyo*) or overcharged (*jitsu*), and this affects our psyche. Dreams can help with diagnosis and play an important part in the healing process. They help you find the right path of action and avoid misfortune, showing energy flowing between the opposites, night and day, yin and yang, heaven and earth, mind and body. We see this particularly through the association of the meridians with the symbols of the Five Processes. For example, when the energy in the Lung

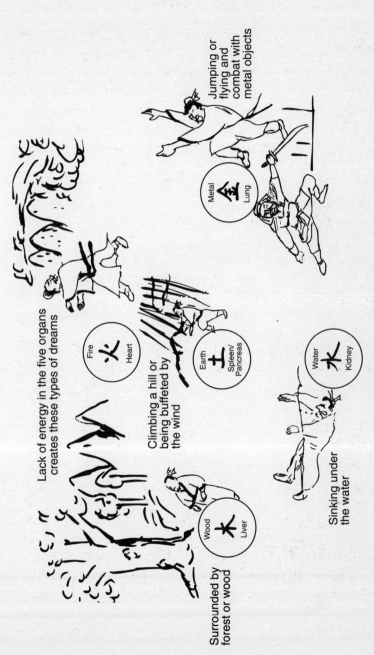

Lack of energy in the five organs creates these types of dreams

Wood — Liver — Surrounded by forest or wood

Fire — Heart — Climbing a hill or being buffeted by the wind

Earth — Spleen/Pancreas

Metal — Lung — Jumping or flying and combat with metal objects

Water — Kidney — Sinking under the water

Five Process Dreams

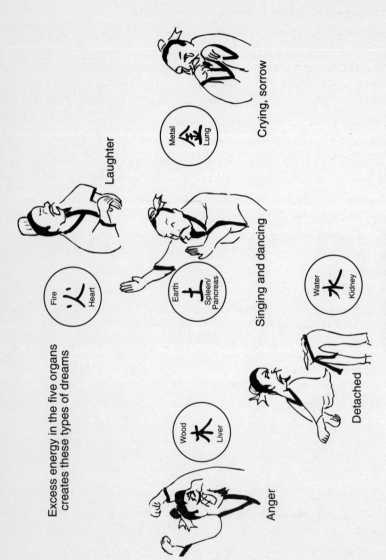

Excess energy in the five organs creates these types of dreams

Laughter

Fire — Heart

Anger

Wood — Liver

Singing and dancing

Earth — Spleen/Pancreas

Metal — Lung

Crying, sorrow

Water — Kidney

Detached

Five Process Dreams

meridian is depleted or empty, we may dream of white objects, or of being cut and seeing blood. In the theory of the Five Processes, the Lung meridian is associated with metal, which is white and cuts things. When the Kidney meridian is empty, weak or depleted, we may dream of drowning or being in a sinking boat. The Kidney meridian is linked with water. If this dream occurs in winter (also associated with water), it could indicate an intense fear of something in the real world. When the Liver meridian is empty or depleted, we may dream of grass growing or, if it is spring, of lying under a big tree, unable to get up. If the Heart meridian is empty or depleted we may dream of extinguishing a fire, for the Heart corresponds to the element fire. When the Spleen-Pancreas is empty or depleted we may dream of being very hungry or, at the end of the summer, of a house or barn being built.

If there is too much rather than too little energy in the meridians, other kinds of symbols appear. If the Lung meridian is overactive, we may dream of crying in intense fear or floating above the ground. Excessive Kidney meridian activity may bring on dreams of our back disintegrating. Frequent angry dreams may indicate an overactive Liver meridian, while dreams of exuberant laughter or shrinking back in fear may come from an overactive Heart meridian. If there is too much energy in the Spleen-Pancreas meridian, we may have dreams of being jovial and exuberant or of feeling burdened and stuck in the body.

THE WAY OF HEAVEN AND EARTH

Like many other phenomena, these dreams are a way to observe the harmony or disharmony of your connection to nature. Recurring dreams in particular can be a warning signal. A patient of mine suffering from depression and terrible fatigue had repeated dreams of flying over a strange dark land towards a hidden goal while tidal waves engulfed the land below. After a few weeks of Shiatsu, the dreams changed. The waves were no longer menacing, the terrifying dark palaces vanished and the dreamer no longer flew. Instead, he was sitting on the ground beside a pleasant brook of sweet flowing water.

I had been working on the Kidney meridian and the Liver meridian of this patient because I noticed that he lacked energy at the very important Kidney source point, which is directly linked to the vital energy of the body as a whole. The Kidney meridian is symbolized as water, while flying indicates too much energy concentrated in the upper part of the body, especially the head. If there is no communication between the flow of heaven's energy in the upper part of the body and the flow of earth's energy in the lower part of the body, the entire yin–yang balance is thrown out of tune. The head accumulates too much yang energy, while yin energy stagnates in the abdomen. It produces symptoms like insomnia, irritability, fatigue, dizziness, cold feet and cold hands.

These dream interpretations, found in *The Yellow Emperor's Classic of Internal Medicine*, are linked with the

theory of the Five Processes. According to this con-
cept, heaven gives virtue and the power to command
love and respect (*toku*) to the earth. When it functions
properly, wisdom flourishes and guides the way to a
long and fruitful life. Our dreams and our sickness are
ways to keep in tune with this Way, if we learn to listen
to them.

3

The Eight Extraordinary Meridians

Unlike traditional Shiatsu, Essential Shiatsu is particularly focused on the role of the Eight Extraordinary Meridians. Despite providing relief from a wide variety of ailments, these eight meridians are not included in most classical descriptions of energy circulation in the Twelve Principal Meridians (although they are mentioned in Japanese translations of *The Yellow Emperor's Classic of Internal Medicine*) and many mysteries still surround them. This is perhaps the first time they have been clearly described.

The job of the Extraordinary Meridians is to absorb and control the abnormal flow of energy from the Principal channels, making them crucial in the body's reaction to malfunction and disease. They use points included in the path of the Principal Meridians, but they connect them in a very different way.

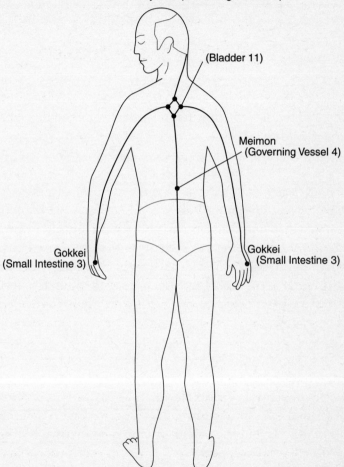

Hiyakue (Governing Vessel 19)

(Bladder 11)

Meimon
(Governing Vessel 4)

Gokkei
(Small Intestine 3)

Gokkei
(Small Intestine 3)

Governing Vessel

THE GOVERNING VESSEL

The Governing Vessel meridian circulates yang energy throughout the body. If it is blocked, this energy does not circulate. This causes stagnation in the extremities, cold hands, cold feet and numbness.

The Governing Vessel originates between the anus and the genital organs and follows the line of the vertebrae to the upper front teeth. It has a connection with the Bladder meridian (the *Fumon* point) that is very important in combating negative energy. If yang energy does not circulate freely on the surface of the body, negative energy can easily penetrate, causing flu and colds. The Governing Vessel and its circulation of yang energy also connect with the right and left kidneys at the *Jinyu* point between lumbar vertebrae two and three. It energizes the kidneys, whose function includes hormonal actions and purification of the blood. These are the elements of fire and water that are fundamental to the life force.

THE CONCEPTION VESSEL

The Conception Vessel meridian circulates yin energy. Chronic ailments are usually associated with stagnation of this energy, so if it can be reactivated the problem will disappear.

The Conception Vessel starts between the anus and the genital organs and continues up along the median line of the body, going around the mouth and ending at the first point of the Stomach meridian,

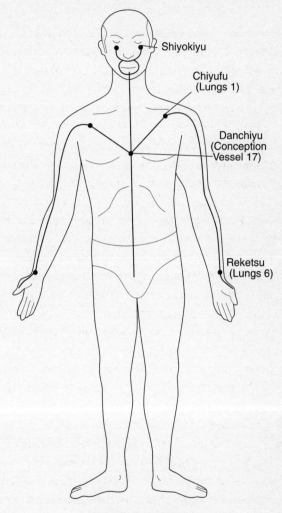

Shiyokiyu

Chiyufu
(Lungs 1)

Danchiyu
(Conception
Vessel 17)

Reketsu
(Lungs 6)

Conception Vessel

Shiyokiyu. It has a very close connection with the Kidney and the Through-going meridians. It is also connected to the Lung meridian at Lung point 1 (*Chiyufu*) and the Conception Vessel at the point *Danchiyu*.

The Conception Vessel regulates all yin meridians. All irregular or abnormal yin energy ends up in the Conception Vessel, which is where we find the stagnant yin energy that causes chronic disease. Yang energy that comes from the Governing Vessel and the right kidney is needed to activate this stagnant yin energy. It battles against negative energy in the defence of the immune system.

The Conception Vessel can liberate potential energy hidden in the body. It connects with the famous *Kikai* point below the navel that is used in martial arts as the foundation of a strong energy field.

THE YANG ANKLE VESSEL

The Yang Ankle Vessel meridian is closely connected to the Governing Vessel. It is associated with the eyes and the yang energy necessary for sight that we use throughout the day.

The Yang Ankle Vessel starts from outside the ankle and follows the external line of the Bladder meridian. It connects with Gall Bladder Point 29 (*Kiyoriyo*), moves along the second line of the Bladder meridian to Point 37 (*Fubun*) and connects with Large Intestine Points 15 and 16. It then connects with the Stomach meridian at Stomach Point 9 (*Jingei*) and follows it until the first

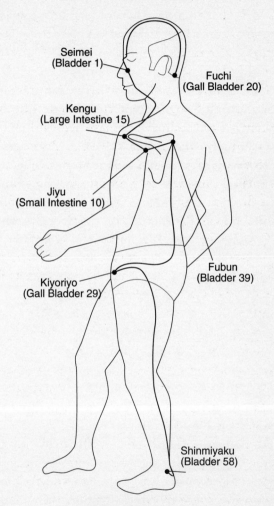

Seimei
(Bladder 1)

Fuchi
(Gall Bladder 20)

Kengu
(Large Intestine 15)

Jiyu
(Small Intestine 10)

Kiyoriyo
(Gall Bladder 29)

Fubun
(Bladder 39)

Shinmiyaku
(Bladder 58)

Yang Ankle Vessel

Stomach point, where it connects with the first point of the Bladder meridian. It follows the Bladder meridian around the head and ends at Gall Bladder Point 20 (*Fuchi*).

The Yang Ankle Vessel meridian is a complex mixture of yang meridians but centres mainly on the Bladder meridian. It follows the outside line of the Bladder meridian along the back. The first line of this meridian, which is linked to the Governing Vessel, is connected with physiological symptoms. The second line, the Yang Ankle Vessel circulation, is connected with psychological symptoms. The first line points at acute problems; the second at much more chronic ones.

THE YIN ANKLE VESSEL

The Yin Ankle Vessel meridian is closely linked to the Conception Vessel and to the eyes when they are closed in sleep. It facilitates the cleaning of toxins from our inner organs. When we are awake, yang energy is active on the surface of our bodies. It concentrates in the eyes, moving through the three yang meridians (Stomach, Gall Bladder and Bladder) that connect the eyes and the feet. The movement of the feet stimulates the eyes. This activates the left brain, which is linked with analytical thought and organization. At night all this yang energy is diverted through the Yin Ankle Vessel into a deeper layer of the body to clear out internal toxins, leaving us recharged with fresh energy so we wake restored.

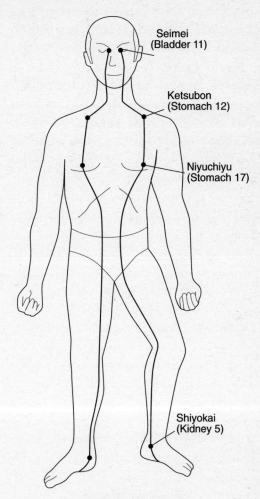

Seimei
(Bladder 11)

Ketsubon
(Stomach 12)

Niyuchiyu
(Stomach 17)

Shiyokai
(Kidney 5)

Yin Ankle Vessel

The Yin Ankle Vessel meridian follows the Kidney
meridian except in the chest area, where it is connected
to the Stomach meridian. It starts from Kidney Point 5
(*Shiyokai*), follows the Stomach meridian until the
Stomach Point (*Ketsubon*), then joins the Through-
going Vessel in the neck. It ends at the first point of the
Bladder meridian. The regulator point is Kidney Point
5 (*Shiyokai*). The Yin Ankle Vessel is closely linked to
the Conception Vessel and thus plays a part in regulating yin body movements. Its activity is linked to the
closing of the eyes and the yin energy activated during
rest. It acts as a counterbalance to the Yang Ankle
Vessel.

THE BELT VESSEL

The Belt Vessel meridian has a short path of circulation. It starts at Liver Point 13 (*Shiyomon*), joins Gall
Bladder Point 26 (*Taimiyoku*), goes around the stomach to Governing Vessel Point 4 (*Meimon*) and enters
the back between lumbar vertebrae two and three. It
then follows the path of the Gall Bladder meridian.
Its regulating point is Gall Bladder Point 4
(*Rinkiyu*).

The Belt Vessel meridian connects yin and yang
meridians and has a strong balancing effect. It is linked
with back problems, lumbar problems, sciatica and
lumbago.

Imbalances of energy flow in our body occur
inevitably as a result of the changing seasons, the
food we eat and the difficulties and psychological

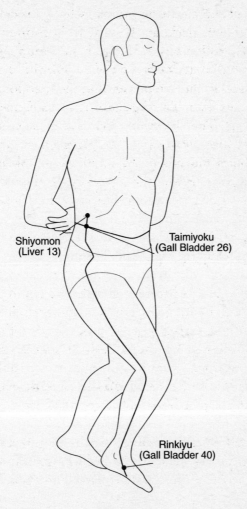

Shiyomon
(Liver 13)

Taimiyoku
(Gall Bladder 26)

Rinkiyu
(Gall Bladder 40)

Belt Vessel

tensions we face in life. The Belt Vessel meridian helps us deal with these imbalances. Yang energy is more available during the day, while yin energy is more available at night, so a person with little yang energy can do exercises with these meridians during the day to benefit from the maximum exposure to natural yang energy.

THE THROUGH-GOING VESSEL

Like the Conception Vessel, the Through-going Vessel meridian begins between the anus and the genital organs. It is closely linked to women's menstrual cycles and works with the Conception Vessel to balance the circulation of hormones. The Through-going Vessel is also involved with introducing inherited energy (from the Kidney) and acquired energy (from the Spleen-Pancreas meridian) to strengthen the body's immune system.

The Through-going Vessel meridian starts in the same place as the Conception Vessel. It crosses the Stomach meridian at Point 30 (*Kishiyo*) and joins the Conception Vessel at the mouth. It then turns downward, moving between the Spleen-Pancreas and Kidney meridians to the knee. There it connects with Kidney Point 10 (*Yinkoku*), moves along the Spleen-Pancreas meridian and ends at the important Spleen-Pancreas Point 4 (*Koson*).

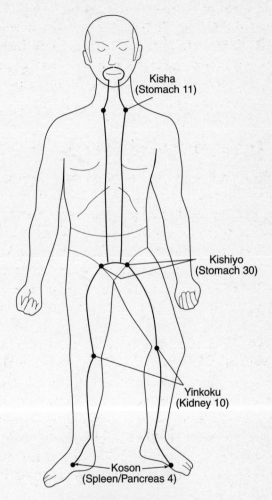

Kisha
(Stomach 11)

Kishiyo
(Stomach 30)

Yinkoku
(Kidney 10)

Koson
(Spleen/Pancreas 4)

Through-going Vessel

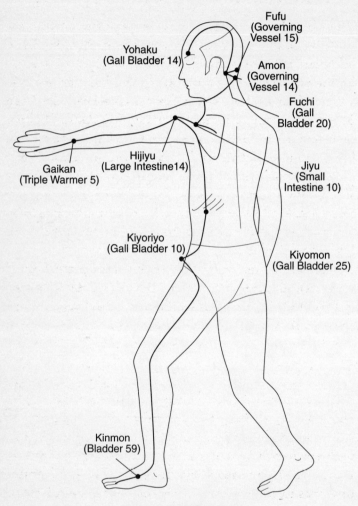

Fufu
(Governing
Vessel 15)

Yohaku
(Gall Bladder 14)

Amon
(Governing
Vessel 14)

Fuchi
(Gall
Bladder 20)

Hijiyu
(Large Intestine14)

Jiyu
(Small
Intestine 10)

Gaikan
(Triple Warmer 5)

Kiyoriyo
(Gall Bladder 10)

Kiyomon
(Gall Bladder 25)

Kinmon
(Bladder 59)

Yang Linking Vessel

THE YANG LINKING VESSEL

The Yang Linking Vessel has perhaps the most complicated course of all the Extraordinary Meridians. It connects all the yang meridians and plays a very important role in correct posture and balance.

The Yang Linking Vessel starts from Bladder Point 59 (*Kinmon*) and immediately joins the Gall Bladder meridian. After Gall Bladder Point 25 (*Kiyomon*), it follows a unique path until it joins Large Intestine Point 14 (*Hijiyu*) and Small Intestine Point 10 (*Jiyu*). It continues on to connect with Triple Warmer Point 15 (*Tenriyo*), Gall Bladder Point 21 (*Kensei*), Governing Vessel Point 14 (*Amon*) and 15 (*Fufu*) and Gall Bladder Point 13 (*Honshin*).

The regulating point is Triple Warmer Point 5 (*Gaikan*), located in the wrist. Like the Belt meridian, with which it is closely linked, it circulates mainly through the Gall Bladder meridian.

THE YIN LINKING VESSEL

The Yin Linking Vessel works with the Through-going Vessel to keep the yin meridians in balance. It starts at Kidney Point 9 (*Chikushin*), follows the Kidney meridian to the knee and joins the Spleen-Pancreas meridian. There it splits, one line going upwards to connect with the Conception Vessel at the neck, the other joining the Heart Constrictor meridian in the arm. The regulating point is Heart Constrictor Point 6 (*Naikan*).

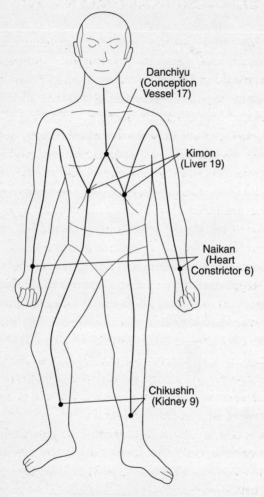

Danchiyu
(Conception
Vessel 17)

Kimon
(Liver 19)

Naikan
(Heart
Constrictor 6)

Chikushin
(Kidney 9)

Yin Linking Vessel

PRINCIPAL MERIDIANS AND EXTRAORDINARY MERIDIANS

Technically we distinguish the Twelve Principal Meridians and the organs they influence from the Eight Extraordinary Meridians and their organs (Brain, Spinal Cord, Bones, Blood Vessels, Gall Bladder and Uterus). The Principal Meridians are overtly or *directly* connected to the organs they influence, whereas the Extraordinary Meridians are covertly or *indirectly* connected to the organs they influence, though their effect is just as powerful. In fact the organs influenced by the Extraordinary Meridians are themselves called 'abnormal' or 'particular'. They are completely paradoxical, looking passive but functioning actively. Their role is ambiguous.

As a group, all these particular organs are related to how we keep our balance and adapt to change. Many of them are interconnected through the Kidney and Gall Bladder meridians. The Brain, the Spinal Cord and the Bones are nourished by the Kidney meridian, while the Gall Bladder is nourished by the Gall Bladder meridian. The Conception Vessel and the Through-going Vessel meridians nourish the Uterus. The Blood Vessels are nourished by the Heart meridian.

All these organs are involved with change and adjusting the balance. The Gall Bladder deserves special mention, for it acts as one of the Principal Meridians too. Unlike the five other organs connected to the Extraordinary Meridians, organs that deal with impure material, the contents of the Gall Bladder, its bile, is 'pure'. It has no foreign matter in it. This is why *The Yellow Emperor's Classic of Internal Medicine* emphasizes the important role of the Gall Bladder in judging and decision-making.

The Brain and the Spinal Cord play active roles in co-ordinating movement, maintaining the agility and mobility necessary to react to sudden change. The Gall Bladder plays a part here, too, helping to maintain balance, both physically and emotionally. The Blood Vessels aid and accompany all these sudden changes of direction. The organs connected with the Extraordinary Meridians all are there to help us adapt to change and keep our balance.

---

8 Extraordinary Vessels
+
6 Particular Inner Organs

---

8 Extraordinary Vessels

- Governing Vessel (yang)
- Conception Vessel (yin)
- Belt Vessel (yang)
- Through-going Vessel (yin)
- Yin Ankle Vessel (yin)
- Yang Ankle Vessel (yang)
- Yin Linking Vessel (yin)
- Yang Linking Vessel (yang)

6 Particular Inner Organs

- Brain
- Spinal Cord
- Bones
- Blood Vessels
- Gall Bladder
- Uterus

Table of Vessels and Organs

YIN AND YANG IN THE EXTRAORDINARY MERIDIANS

Meridians have either yin or yang qualities and thus different functions and different things affect them. Wind, cold, heat, humidity and dryness affect the yang meridians. They are vulnerable when the hair follicles are loosened or the skin is broken. As long as your skin is intact, the yang meridians will protect you. Their job is to prevent negative energy from entering the body.

The yin meridians maintain the internal regulating system, sustain the yang meridians and protect the body from within. They are attacked by internal problems, such as bad diet or too much sex. Traditional oriental medicine says too much sex weakens the Kidneys and affects the immune system. Sexual behaviour is linked to the Kidney meridian, while metabolism is linked to the Stomach and Spleen-Pancreas meridians, which are responsible for producing nourishing and defensive energy. These two systems are the backbone of our self-regulating or immune system.

The yin meridians are protected by the yang meridians, and in turn nourish the yang meridians. The Belt Vessel, which circles the lumbar region, is the only meridian that connects all yin and yang meridians. This connection is very important. The Belt Vessel connects with the Governing Vessel Point (*Meimon*), crosses the two Bladder meridian lines (*Jinyu* and *Shishitsu*), then crosses the great transversal of the Spleen-Pancreas and the Kidney meridians to join the Conception Vessel. The zone of the Belt Vessel includes the Kidney,

Conception Vessel and Governing Vessel meridians. The Kidneys play a key function in this interchange. The right Kidney is linked with fire and yang, the left Kidney with water and yin. Fire and water are the elements that create the life force and make the movement of energy possible. The Governing Vessel (right Kidney) and the Conception Vessel (left Kidney) represent these functions.

4

Everyday Work with the Extraordinary Meridians

Exercises connected with each of the Eight Extraordinary Meridians can give everyone access to their healing energy. They can be done by anyone with a bit of will and endurance, and the benefits in health and the feeling of connection and well-being can be truly spectacular. The exercises are particularly good for those suffering from sleeping problems, stress or fatigue.

Do these exercises every morning and evening. The spirit of concentration is important. Morning exercise lets you draw on the rising energy of nature, while evening exercise helps you rid your body of the fatigue and negative energy accumulated during the day. Do not do the exercises after a meal or an operation, or if you have a fever.

Some of these exercises are difficult, even for the young and supple, but perfection is not the goal. The essential thing is to relax your muscles and do the positions without strain. If you experience discomfort, stop

and try another exercise. If you find a blocked meridian, spend more time working with it, breathing slowly
and steadily. If you do not have enough time to do all
eight exercises, concentrate on the two most important:
the Governing Vessel and the Conception Vessel.

Remember that breathing is important. When doing
the exercises, breathe in while you are stretching and
breathe out after maximum extension. Exhalation is a
vital part of the exercise. Unless you exhale calmly and
smoothly, the next inhalation will be constricted. Then
your breathing will block the flow of energy in the
meridians rather than letting it flow smoothly.

THE REGULATING POINTS

Each Extraordinary Meridian has a central regulating
or governing point that controls the flow of energy
throughout. These points are all located near the ankle
or wrist, parts of the body that are constantly in motion.
You can start your exercise session by pressing these
points.

Governing Vessel: Small Intestine point (*Gokkei*)
Conception Vessel: Lung point (*Reketsu*)
Yang Ankle Vessel: Bladder point (*Shinmiyaku*)
Yin Ankle Vessel: Kidney point (*Shiyokai*)
Belt Vessel: Gall Bladder point (*Rinkiyu*)
Through-going Vessel: Spleen-Pancreas point (*Koson*)
Yang Linking Vessel: Triple Warmer point (*Gaikan*)
Yin Linking Vessel: Heart Constrictor point (*Naikan*)

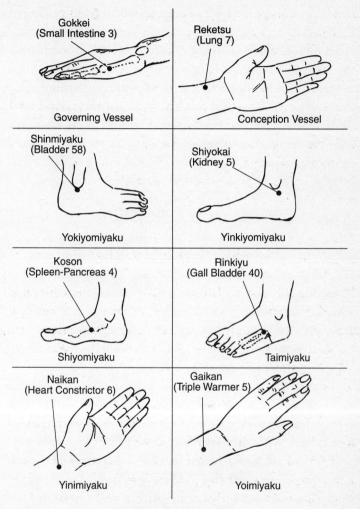

Gokkei
(Small Intestine 3)

Reketsu
(Lung 7)

Governing Vessel

Conception Vessel

Shinmiyaku
(Bladder 58)

Shiyokai
(Kidney 5)

Yokiyomiyaku

Yinkiyomiyaku

Koson
(Spleen-Pancreas 4)

Rinkiyu
(Gall Bladder 40)

Shiyomiyaku

Taimiyaku

Naikan
(Heart Constrictor 6)

Gaikan
(Triple Warmer 5)

Yinimiyaku

Yoimiyaku

Regulating Points

Those who are physically disabled or have become stiff can also use the regulating points of the Eight Extraordinary Meridians very effectively. Before doing the exercises, prepare and loosen the body by applying pressure to these points or having someone else do it for you. It is important to acquire the habit of stimulating these points every day. You will soon notice the improvement in your muscle flexibility. If the muscles are not regularly stretched and exercised they tighten up and can become permanently stiff.

BASIC EXERCISES

In doing these exercises, give yourself enough time to feel at ease, and wear comfortable, loose clothing. Try to empty your mind of your daily preoccupations and simply give yourself to the exercise. Breathe deeply and regularly and do not try to force the stretches. As you actively relax into the positions, you will find them both enjoyable and invigorating.

The most important basic exercise works on the Governing Vessel. It is easy to do and you will feel its effects quite quickly. If you are stiff or not used to exercise, begin with this exercise alone.

There is no fixed order for these postures. You can start anywhere you like. However the order listed on pages 72–4 is particularly helpful in strengthening the immune system.

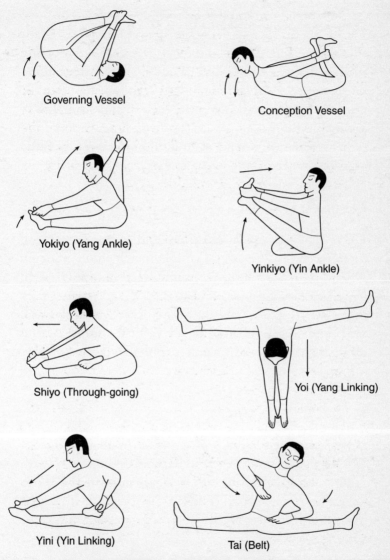

Governing Vessel

Conception Vessel

Yokiyo (Yang Ankle)

Yinkiyo (Yin Ankle)

Shiyo (Through-going)

Yoi (Yang Linking)

Yini (Yin Linking)

Tai (Belt)

Extraordinary Meridian Stretches

GOVERNING VESSEL

Lie on your back, take hold of the soles of your feet and rock back and forth, rolling your spine against the floor. Keep your neck soft. Do not let your chin stick out. All the effort involved should come from your lower abdomen. Start from your coccyx and gently roll up to the first dorsals. Avoid rolling on your neck. Breathe normally.

CONCEPTION VESSEL

Lie on your stomach and take hold of your feet. Roll forward and backward on your stomach gently, rocking on the centre. Breathe normally. If you cannot reach your feet, imagine you are holding them. Perfect posture is not the aim. Visualize the position and follow its movement possibilities. This exercise should not be done by people with back problems or by women during a menstrual period.

YANG ANKLE VESSEL

Hold your big toe with your thumb and forefingers. Lift your leg and stretch it outwards. Follow it with your eyes. Keep your other leg firmly on the floor. Inhale as you lengthen your leg and exhale as it returns to centre. Repeat with the other leg.

YIN ANKLE VESSEL

Sit in the *Seiza* position, with one leg bent back along your thigh, close to your body. Inhale, hold your back straight and stretch forward to the extended foot. Raise it slowly in front of you as high as you can. Repeat five or six times on each side.

THROUGH-GOING VESSEL

Sit and place one foot on the thigh of the opposite leg. Stretch forward and grasp the extended foot with both hands. Inhale, hold your back straight and stretch your body forward to the extended foot. Repeat five or six times on each side.

BELT VESSEL

Sit with your legs apart, placing one hand on your hip and the other high on your rib cage. Inhale and lean toward the side where you are holding your hip. Repeat five or six times on each side. Then put both hands on your hips and make circles with your body, moving from the base of your spine, thirty times in each direction.

YANG LINKING VESSEL

Open your legs as wide as you can. Place your hands

on the floor in front of you. Slide your hands slowly forward and, keeping your back straight, let your body follow them forward. Inhale as you go towards the floor. Stop when it interferes with your breathing.

YIN LINKING VESSEL

Sit and fold your right foot on to your left thigh. Hold your foot in place, reaching behind your back with your right hand and grasping it. Keep your spine straight. Reach forward and grab your left foot with your left hand. This is a difficult posture. Simply feel the movements of energy as much as you can. If you are stiff, do not be discouraged. Breathe gently and rhythmically and do what you can. If you can imagine the movement, your body will follow. Repeat five or six times on each side.

5

Treatment

THE BASIC DIAGNOSIS

The basic function of the Eight Extraordinary Meridians is to adjust the changing influence of yin and yang energies in the various parts of the body and the various Principal Meridians. The practitioner can use these eight meridians and the points associated with them to get a clear picture of what is going on in the patient's body and mind.

As we have seen, the Essential Shiatsu symbol shows the movement of yin and yang. Yin energy descends from heaven to earth. Yang energy ascends from earth to heaven. The diagram portrays the interaction or symbolic marriage of yin and yang through the elements of fire and water. These movements are fundamental to the practice of Shiatsu.

When we treat people, the basic step in making a diagnosis is touching the vital energy pulsation point,

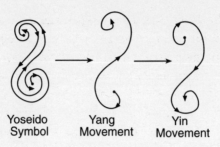

Yoseido   Yang   Yin
Symbol   Movement   Movement

Shiatsu Symbol

Kikaitanden, one and a half to two thumbs below the navel. This is where vital energy, product of the connection of yin and yang, rests. It gives us an overall diagnosis of health, particularly the state of the immune system. If this point is calm and stable, no matter how dreadful the symptoms may be an eventual cure is certain. If it is unstable, shaky or empty, the road to health will be long and difficult.

If a patient's *Kikaitanden* is empty, we must try to fill it. This can be a protracted process. It can take a month or more before you can feel the energy recharging. The more chronic the problem, the more time is required. Miracles do happen, just not overnight.

Once the practitioner has noted the patient's basic energy level, then feel the balance of heaven and earth energies. A hand is placed on Stomach meridian point 25, two thumbs away from the navel. This point is called *Tensu* or Heaven's Axis. It shows you the movement of energy between heaven and earth in the individual, for it is a bridge between them, and gives you a sense of the person's overall well-being or lack of it. When the flow or interchange of energy is harmonious, the point will feel firm but supple. When there is blockage, it feels stiff and tight. When people have headaches or sleeping problems, you will find a tight knot here.

DOCTORS AND DIVINERS

If you think that the purpose of medicine is simply the curing of disease, you are like a fortune-teller who feels he or she must always be objectively right. A doctor and a diviner do have a deep connection, but neither one of them should be judged on the standard of being 'right'. Things are much more subtle than that. The *sho* or 'proof of the diagnosis' is more than a simple coincidence of diagnosis and symptoms. It has to do with what Japanese call *shinsen-jitsu*, understanding how to preserve the human vital force. Similarly the *shiyoho*, the 'prescription of medication appropriate to the symptoms', must be understood in terms of the individual case – the individual person – rather than the statistical cure of a generalized disease.

Oriental medicine, at its best, is more than a cure of disease. It looks at the life of each person and the place of the 'disease' in that life. This means a 'disease' is different for each person that has it. This is the kind of wholeness we see as our ideal. The diagnosis of a doctor is much like an oracle at a Shinto shrine or an *I Ching* consultation; it depends on who is there, on who is asking the question, and who is giving the answer.

When you diagnose, never forget this. You are part of the equation, and each diagnosis is unique.

ABDOMINAL DIAGNOSIS

Another very significant diagnostic method involves the abdomen or *hara*, an important term in Japanese. It means the field of harvest, source of the energy that can replenish people.

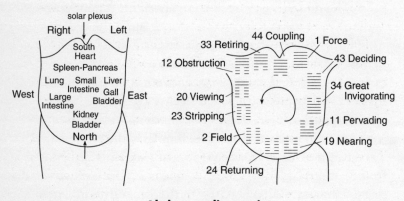

Abdomen diagnosis

As you can see, each internal organ is thought to have a specific place on the abdomen. The directions, the twelve Chinese 'year animals' and diagrams (*gua*) from the *I Ching* showing the rise and fall of yang energy are associated with these points. East shows the rise of yang energy and spring; south shows the zenith of yang energy and summer; west the decline of yang, the rise of yin and autumn; north shows maximum yin and winter.

The organ positions are very important, and have psychological as well as physiological meanings. The Heart holds the *shin* that contains a person's unifying personality. The Spleen-Pancreas holds the *shyu*, a person's mental reflection or deep thought, the intellectual capacity to reason things out. The Kidney holds *shi*, the libido, an instinctive drive towards self-preservation, sex and desire. Ideally these three have a triadic relationship, where noble thought (*shin*) combines with practical mind (*shyu*) to curtail instinctive drive (*shi*) and arrive at a concrete realization.

The abdominal region represents extreme yin, and thus is particularly important in diagnosis. Such a diagnosis, however, does not mean detecting disease or dysfunction in the organs, but refers to a much more subtle condition that precedes dysfunction, the emptiness (*kyo*) or excess (*jitsu*) of energy flow in the organs. This relies heavily on intuition and demands concentration and the right attitude. Shiatsu is an art of feeling the wholeness of a person rather than separating and dissecting individual symptoms.

DISHARMONY AND LACK OF ENERGY

Treating this lack of energy, which reflects a disharmony between heaven and earth energies, is a fairly simple procedure. Here are two Shiatsu treatments and an exercise that can help people with these problems.

PULLING THE LEGS

The first treatment involves simply pulling the patient's legs toward you. Place your middle fingers on the sides of the patient's feet at Kidney Point 3 (*Taikei*), the source point of the Kidney meridian. Take hold of the feet and pull the legs toward you gently.

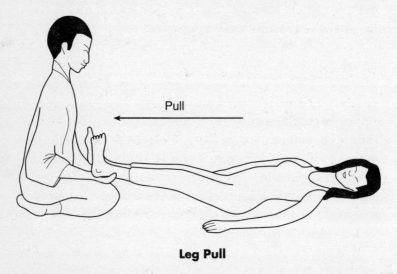

Pull

Leg Pull

When you do this, you must not pull too much or too little. The pulling must be very subtle to be effective. The key point is to inhale as you pull and to exhale slowly from the abdomen as you release the pressure. When this is done correctly, the person receiving treatment feels an agreeable tension around the *Kikaitanden* area. Maintain the pull for five to ten minutes. If the patient has a severe lack of energy it is possible to pull for up to thirty minutes. You must, however, get used to the sitting position the Japanese call *Seiza* (see illustration). To take this position, fold your legs under you. Arrange your right foot, and then put your left foot on top of it. The right foot is a symbol of yin and the left a symbol of yang. So heaven (yang) is placed higher than earth (yin). This method of pulling on the feet adjusts deficient energy as well as blocked heaven and earth energies. Here the legs and feet are yin parts of the body, so we call this a yin approach.

PULLING THE ARMS

Another effective method is to pull on the patient's arm. Place both hands on the patient's wrist. Put both thumbs together on the Triple Warmer Point 4 (*Yochi*) and press firmly. Pull on the arm gently, and be careful not to hurt the wrist or shoulder. The patient should feel a gentle but focused tension in the *Kikaitanden* area.

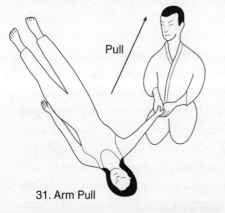

Pull

31. Arm Pull

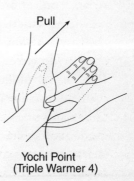

Pull

Yochi Point
(Triple Warmer 4)

Arm Pull

Though both of these methods are quite effective, pulling the arm is more difficult than pulling the leg. Unless you are quite careful, the patient may feel you are pinching or squeezing. Neither should be done when the patient's joints are painful. Shiatsu is not torture; it should be done in an agreeable and comfortable way. The energy moves at deep levels only when the people involved, patient and practitioner, are fully relaxed. Because these pulling techniques have no violent movements, they are particularly suitable for those whose energy is fragile, who are in precarious health, bed-ridden or elderly.

THE STOMACH POINT

Stomach meridian Point 30 (*Kishiyo*) plays a vital role in taking external energy into the bloodstream. All digestive, absorption and evacuation problems relate to this point, and patients with digestive problems will have a strong, regular pulsation here, accompanied by pain. Almost all problems with digestion and assimilation of food focus on the Stomach and Spleen-Pancreas meridians.

Why do we encounter so many Stomach and Spleen-Pancreas problems? Much of it has to do with the way we lead our lives. We eat foods that are full of preservatives and additives. We keep irregular hours and take inadequate exercise, particularly the vital leg exercise that stimulates and strengthens the Stomach meridian. Because the Stomach and Spleen-Pancreas meridians are so vulnerable to pollutants, we need special exercises to stimulate and balance them. Families can help each other by walking on each other's thighs, an exercise that stimulates all the meridians.

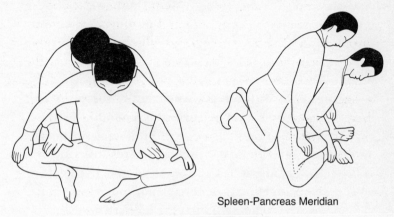

Spleen-Pancreas Meridian

Spleen-Pancreas Stretch

We can use this exercise particularly to stimulate the Spleen-Pancreas meridian. The person receiving the treatment must be quite supple in the hips. In the illustration we see someone who can let his legs open completely to lie flat on the ground. We can promote this flexibility by pressing the *Kishiyo* point with the palms of our hands. The more we do this, the more supple the joints become.

THE TWELVE PRINCIPAL POINTS

After you have gained an overall picture of the patient's vital energy, you can examine his health in more detail by looking at the source point (*gen*) of each of the Twelve Principal Meridians. Innate and acquired energies combine at these points to establish the body's immune system, our capacity to respond to our environment. All the source points are found at the wrists and ankles, which suggests they have a profound influence on the flexibility of the body.

Palpate each of these points carefully to see if they have a strong pulsation or current. Generally, a strong superficial pulsation indicates an abundance of energy, and weak interior pulsation indicates insufficient energy flow. Linger on the spot to see if the flow changes. Changes can occur, sometimes slowly and sometimes very quickly. Different colours may appear on the points. Blue usually means pain; black shows pressure due to a cyst or tumour; white means cold; a mixture of yellow and red shows heat. When red and white are mixed, there is a combination of hot and cold. Also note dryness or sweating at each point. Cold moisture indicates excessive yin; hot dryness indicates excessive yang. Sometimes a particular smell may come from a point.

All of the twelve source points are closely linked with the organs of the body and offer valuable clues to how they are functioning. If any of these points are blocked, showing no strong pulse, we can assume that the corresponding organs are not functioning correctly.

The Twelve Source Points

Lung Meridian	Large Intestine Meridian	Stomach Meridian	Spleen-Pancreas Meridian	Heart Meridian	Small Intestine Meridian
Taien (lung 9)	Gokoku (large intestine 4)	Shiyoyo (stomach 42)	Taihaku (spleen-pancreas 3)	Shinma (heart 7)	Wankotsu (small intestine 4)
Bladder Meridian	Kidney Meridian	Heart-Constrictor Meridian	Triple Warmer Meridian	Gall Bladder Meridian	Liver Meridian
Kiyokotsu (bladder 60)	Taikei (kidney 3)	Dairiyo (heart constrictor 7)	Yochi (triple warmer 4)	Kiyukiyo (gall bladder 39)	Taisho (liver 3)

WORKING ON THE NECK

The neck offers another important opportunity to understand what is going on in the body. The head is the most yang part of the body, as the chest is the most yin. The hands are said to be yin functionaries as the feet are yang functionaries. Energy flows between the chest and head through the neck, which connects them to the arms and hands. All the yang hand meridians terminate on the face by passing through the neck, while yang meridians that begin in the face pass through the neck to the feet. Anything connected with head problems – deteriorating memory, stoppages in the nose, poor eyesight, paralysis, epilepsy, or insomnia – is connected to the neck.

First carefully inspect each of the Principal Meridians that run through the neck: Small Intestine, Large Intestine, Triple Warmer, Stomach, Bladder and Gall Bladder (see illustration). Inspect, too, the yin meridians that run to or through the neck to the head. Even the most yang part of the body (the head) has a yin meridian running through it, the Liver meridian. It joins the Governing Vessel at Point 19 (*Hiyakue*). The yin meridians of the Pancreas, Heart and Kidney all join the back of the neck. Persistent coughs can be traced here to weakness in the Kidney or the related Spleen-Pancreas meridian.

The neck is supported by seven cervical vertebrae that move and turn the head through the intricately twined neck muscles. These deep neck muscles sometimes cause the vertebrae to slip their discs, the pads of

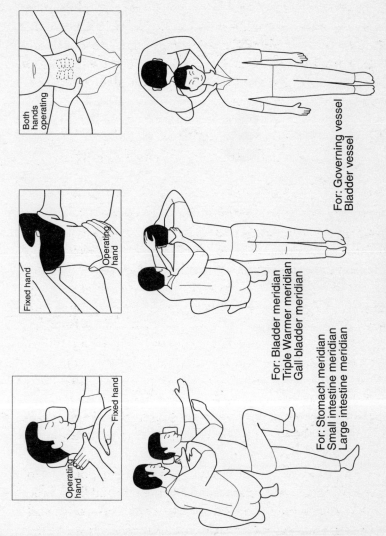

Operating hand

Fixed hand

For: Stomach meridian
Small intestine meridian
Large intestine meridian

Fixed hand

Operating hand

For: Bladder meridian
Triple Warmer meridian
Gall bladder meridian

Both hands operating

For: Governing vessel
Bladder vessel

Head and Neck

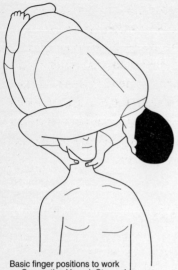

Basic finger positions to work
on Conception Vessel, Stomach,
Small Intestine and Bladder
meridians and the Governing Vessel

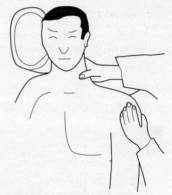

Basic neck position to work on the
Stomach, Large Intestine, Triple Warmer,
Gall Bladder and Bladder meridians

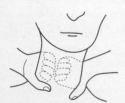

Finger position for working on the
Governing and Bladder Vessel meridians

Head and Neck

cartilage between them or become misaligned. Specific organs of the body nourish the neck muscles, so if someone is suffering from a misarranged vertebra we can find the root cause in the malfunctioning of an organ of the body. Similarly, if someone is suffering from a stiff neck and cannot turn his head, we read it as a message from nature telling the person to stay quiet and rest rather than going immediately to work. Turning the head symbolizes decision-making and stress, which creates tension in the body.

BACK PAINS

Back problems such as lumbago and sciatica usually appear in the lumbar region, which is circled and governed by the Belt Vessel. Chiropractors are kept quite busy trying to deal with these conditions directly but the problems themselves are caused by blocks in the Stomach meridian associated with lack of exercise, too much stimulation through tea, coffee, cigarettes and alcohol, and an unbalanced diet. The Belt Vessel stretching exercise shown on page 73 can help most of these disorders, even serious disc hernia.

PSYCHOLOGICAL PROBLEMS

Psychological problems are closely connected with the left side of the first and second cervical vertebrae. Traumatic experiences can be seen on these vertebrae, while chronic depression can be felt in the neck and the top of the head. Neck complications are linked with other parts of the body through the Gall Bladder, Liver, Bladder and Triple Warmer meridians. When the cervical region is deformed, it blocks the circulation of the Governing Vessel, which can lead to all sorts of psychological abnormalities.

DEVIATION OF THE VERTEBRAE

A person's posture and the way in which the spine supports the posture give us further indications of health or sickness. Deviations in the lumbar spine and the thorax can block the circulation of energy into the Governing Vessel, which runs along the line of the spine.

Usually the deviation of a vertebra can be directly traced to the Governing Vessel meridian and the Bladder meridian that runs next to it. The Bladder meridian has two parallel tracks that run from the first thoracic vertebra down to the fifth lumbar vertebra. The internal line, the one closest to the Governing Vessel, has a physiological effect and influences the internal organs. The external Bladder line has a close association with the psychological functioning of the patient.

In persistent problems, the points corresponding to the problems will often shift from the internal line to the external or psychological one. I have often observed this phenomenon. For example, soon after a physiological problem was resolved, a patient complained that the

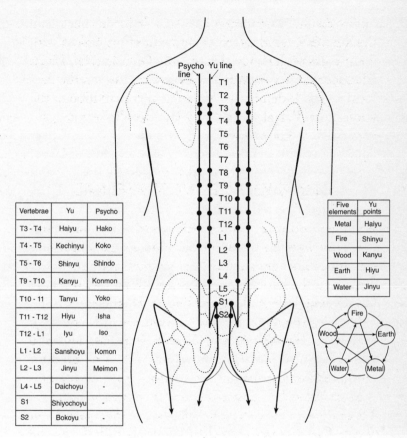

Vertebrae	Yu	Psycho
T3 - T4	Haiyu	Hako
T4 - T5	Kechinyu	Koko
T5 - T6	Shinyu	Shindo
T9 - T10	Kanyu	Konmon
T10 - 11	Tanyu	Yoko
T11 - T12	Hiyu	Isha
T12 - L1	Iyu	Iso
L1 - L2	Sanshoyu	Komon
L2 - L3	Jinyu	Meimon
L4 - L5	Daichoyu	-
S1	Shiyochoyu	-
S2	Bokoyu	-

Five elements	Yu points
Metal	Haiyu
Fire	Shinyu
Wood	Kanyu
Earth	Hiyu
Water	Jinyu

Spinal Points

pain had returned. There was, however, no tension at all at the point corresponding to the physiological problem. When I looked at the corresponding point on the psychological line, however, I found a very tight, hard, crystal-like knot. I concluded that there must be a significant psychological dimension to the problem.

In oriental medicine, we make no separation between mind and body and try to consider the patient as a whole. *The Yellow Emperor's Classic of Internal Medicine* tells us that every organ has a psychic entity connected to it. The Heart has the *shin*; the Liver has the *kon*; the Kidney has the *sei*; the Lung has the *haku*; and the Spleen-Pancreas has the *I*. Each manifestation of psychic behaviour is influenced by one of these spirits. Excessive anger, for instance, is caused by the *kon* and can seriously damage the Liver. The spirits of the organs are directed by the *shin* of the Heart, which is like the conductor of a symphony who synchronizes the overall sound of the music. The *shin* tries to integrate the entire personality.

The psychological aspects of problems can often be felt between the fifth and sixth thoracic vertebrae. Depressive people will have a concave fifth and sixth vertebrae, as will those with a weak heart. The Governing Vessel also plays an important part, orchestrating both physical and mental well-being.

TREATMENTS USING THE EIGHT EXTRAORDINARY MERIDIANS

WARMING THINGS UP

A Danish man came to see me about his impotence. He had a good professional reputation and worked quite hard. Unlike many people with this problem, he did not drink or smoke heavily. I examined his abdomen and noticed his Liver and Kidney regions were empty of energy. His eyes were deteriorating rapidly, particularly his right eye. In response to my questions, he said that he had a strong desire to make love with a particular woman whom he loves, but he simply could not have an erection, something that frustrated him and his partner.

In oriental medicine, such a desire is linked with the Kidney function, while the actual erection during love-making is connected with the Liver function. Liver and Kidney work side by side to do the work.

This gentleman told me that his work was very difficult and stressful. He had no time to exercise. Sometimes he swam. He ate sweets and, when he was under stress, he ate chocolate cake and drank coffee.

Treatment When I pressed the *Saninko* point (where the Liver, Spleen and Kidney meridians join), it was painful. I worked on the Through-going meridian and the Yin Linking meridian, and connected the regulating point of the Through-going meridian (*Koson*) and the regulating point of the Yin Linking meridian (*Naikan*).

The Heart Constrictor points on his left arm were quite hard and painful, but after I worked on them he felt considerable relief. I told him to do the stretching exercises for the Through-going meridian, the Yin Linking meridian and the Governing meridian each day.

His treatments were two or three times a week at first, then once a week. After two and a half months he was able to have a firm erection. I gave him an exercise to stimulate his testicles and told him to do it in the bathroom each morning to stimulate the circulation of yang energy. I also told him that deep breathing is the key to yang circulation.

Scientists have studied the question of potency and sperm count in men living in the far north. No one has come up with an answer, though lack of light, pollution and stress have been suggested. Southern peoples are not afflicted by this problem so much. Northern people have much less exposure to the sun and spend much more time indoors, so their body energy stagnates. It is natural wisdom to have invented the sauna as a counteractive to this condition.

A sauna offers a way to eliminate the body's built-up toxins. In these cold climates people eat more salty and more fatty foods. Salt and fat seal the body off against cold but, at the same time, impede the circulation of the blood. People in these environments must constantly energize their metabolism and circulation through exercise and sauna. The exercises for the Eight Extraordinary Meridians are ideal, particularly if they are done vigorously and are followed by a hot shower.

STEP BY STEP

I was consulted by a German businessman about his gallstone problem. He was impeccably dressed from head to toe, and maintained that he never drank or ate to excess – no fatty foods, no coffee, and no sweets.

Treatment I examined his abdomen to see where the energy flow was excessive or deficient. His Gall Bladder area was weak, his Spleen-Pancreas had a strong rapid pulse and his Kidney area was empty. He told me that he often felt quite tired between 5 and 7 p.m. This is the Kidney hour, which connects directly to the Gall Bladder.

This man had suffered from gallstones for several years. There were no signs of acute pain at present, but whenever he was stressed and socially overextended the acute signs in the Gall Bladder region showed up. His doctor confirmed he had had several very painful episodes.

In the Five Processes theory, when the wood element of the Gall Bladder weakens, the earth element of the Spleen-Pancreas becomes overactive. It absorbs the water of the Kidney and weakens it. The Kidney in turn further weakens and deactivates the element of wood in the Gall Bladder.

The regulating point of the Belt meridian (*Rinkiyu*) was quite painful, but the regulating point of the Through-going meridian (*Koson*) caused even more excruciating agony. I worked on both meridians, and on key points connected with the Yang Linking meridian and the Yin Linking meridian. After five treatments, the acute pain lessened. I suggested that he could do the meridian stretching exercises every day.

The patient grew less tired each day and discharged his gallstones. In oriental medicine, gallstones are connected with decision-making and perfectionism. Perhaps this gentleman's lifestyle contributed to his affliction. This perfectionism sometimes leaves no place to breathe, like a compact crystal that prohibits anyone a chance to move through it.

The Belt meridian, which I used to cure this man, is very interesting. It has a very short passage in which it connects all the energy meridians that flow through the centre of the body. It connects the Conception Vessel meridian and the Governing meridian, front and back, and all the major organs are found in this area. The Extraordinary Meridians constantly balance the flow of energy, and the Belt meridian is the primary agent for this function, constantly mediating between left and right. People with migraine or gallstones can deal with their problem by stimulating the points involved.

FIRE AND WATER

A seventy-year-old man came to see me complaining of prostate trouble, cold feet and impaired circulation. His eyes ran continually. I palpated his abdomen and found the Kidney region very cold, empty and without resistance, while the Heart area was hard, rigid and painful. He generally felt uncomfortable and op-pressed, and showed a complete lack of energy in the Kidney area and blocked energy around the Heart. In Japanese medicine this is *jiyojitsu kakiyo*, 'upper stiff-ness and lower emptiness'. In my understanding of the *I Ching*, this state is represented by the diagram called *64 Not Yet Fording*, where fire (Heart) and water (Kidney) fail to mix together. This is a very imbal-anced state, as opposed to *63 Already Fording*, which shows fire and water successfully interacting. This is a quite healthy condition often found in martial arts experts.

Treatment Preserving yang energy as long as possible is extremely important. It leads directly to long life and good health. The Extraordinary Meridians are crucial here, especially the Governing Vessel. It has a very close relation with both right and left Kidneys, which signify the water function in the body (left Kidney) and the fire function in the body (right Kidney).

This man's watery eyes were directly linked to the Bladder meridian at the first Bladder point (*Semei*). This connects with the Governing Vessel at the left Kidney, the water sign. It showed excess. The right Kidney, the fire sign, was linked to the bottom of the feet at Kidney Point 1 (*Yusen*).

Yang energy ascends while yin energy descends. Philosophically heaven is the place of yang and earth is the place of yin, and physiologically the eyes are heaven's place and the soles of the feet are earth's place. Inside yang, there is yin; inside yin there is yang, but here all was disrupted. The constant flow of liquid in this man's eyes connected with yin and the left Kidney, and showed too much yin above. The cold feet, which should be warm and dry, reflected the right or fire Kidney and showed too little yang below. Philosophically and physiologically, this was a state of extreme imbalance.

Because of the constricting and slowing effect of yin energy, which acted directly on the prostate, it was of crucial importance to activate yang energy through work on the Governing Vessel meridian. I stimulated all the points on this meridian as well as concentrating on its regulating point (*Gokkei*, Small

Intestine 3). This point, on both sides of the meridian, was completely rigid, like limestone, as were the Governing Vessel points along the spine. This Extraordinary Meridian was the key, for the man was in very deep trouble. I worked with all the points, then told him to do the Governing Vessel stretching exercise at home, as slowly as he needed to do it. I also instructed him to do deep breathing exercises while putting his hands over his abdomen and pushing it out as he exhaled.

He came three times a week for treatment and faithfully did the exercises. After two months, his eyes cleared up, his abdomen began to react directly to touch, and the pressure on his prostate was relieved. The *Gokkei* points (Governing Vessel regulator) became much less sensitive and the muscles of his back and shoulders became more flexible. Though we had not made a young man out of a seventy-year-old citizen, we had at least given him, so to speak, a new lease on life.

WRESTLING WITH LIFE

A forty-year-old Japanese businessman came to see me because he could hardly stand up straight. He was in intense pain. The first day he walked in, he was holding himself together with his hands. He told me that when he had to go down a staircase he felt an intense pain like an electric shock penetrate his abdomen and back. He called it chronic lumbago. As I palpated his abdominal region, he felt intense pain in the Liver region. The right side of his diaphragm was very stiff and uncomfortable, while the Kidney area had a deep strong pulse. When I gently pressed the *Rinkiyu* point (Gall Bladder 40), which is the regulating point of the Belt Vessel, it was so painful he almost leaped into the air.

Treatment This man looked like a sumo wrestler, strong, muscular, dense, aggressive, weighing more than ninety-five kilos. But, he said, even he 'could not bear this kind of pressure'. I gradually understood what the pressure was. This man was a representative in Europe for a major Japanese car manufacturer. His life was a succession of planes, trains, hotels, rented cars and restaurants. He ate and drank heavily, got no exercise, and only walked between a car and an elevator. His body was obviously giving him a very simple message: Either you stop this, or I will cripple you. He wouldn't listen. He tried to keep on, gobbling prescription painkillers and taking shots.

He needed help fast, and that is what the Extraordinary Meridians are there for. I worked carefully on all the Belt Vessel points to disperse the excess energy, concentrating on the *Rinkiyu* or regulating point. It took only two sessions to relieve his pain and start him walking normally again. What a miracle, he said. I told him it was not in the least a miracle: the miracle was the message his body had given him. Acute problems like these are very easy to handle because a healthy body is reacting to imbalanced energy. But the fundamental problem is still there – things are still out of kilter and there is something unspoken and distorted that must be looked after. The Yellow Emperor's text speaks about this. Because this man was oriental, he understood. I showed him the Belt Vessel stretching exercise, a very important Extraordinary Meridian, and told him to come at least ten more times. He did, and he has not had a recurrence of his chronic lumbago.

COLD HANDS, COLD FEET

A Japanese woman pianist came to see me, complaining of great fatigue and lassitude. Her hands and feet were very cold, and she had difficulty sleeping. She had pain in her shoulders and elbows. I soon found out that she had recently had a child. She had breast-fed her child at all hours and, between feeding and a rigorous schedule of concert rehearsals, had had almost no sleep. She was into a cycle of chronic fatigue.

Treatment When I palpated her abdomen, I found the Heart region extremely tense. The Liver and Kidney areas felt empty, and the Spleen and Stomach were very empty indeed. The tense Heart and Solar Plexus were at the centre of her sleep problem. I touched her Heart Source Point (*Shinmon*, Heart 7) which was very, very tense, but the root of the problem came from somewhere else. I had a sudden vision. I saw the Through-going Vessel (*Shiyomiyaku*), which explained that the Kidney, Spleen and Stomach weakness indicated that both acquired and innate energies were lacking. Because she had a child and had to keep working as a pianist, she was no longer up to the enormously stressful demands of playing concert piano.

Here we must look at the situation of our patient. She was a student at a very prestigious conservatory, a position that demanded almost supernormal discipline. Your fate is decided in one performance; you have no second chance. Everything is staked on the Heart meridian, the unifier and co-ordinator. It is the *shin*, the spirit that brings everything together.

I treated this woman by working on the Through-going Vessel (Heart) along with its regulating point (*Koson*, Spleen-Pancreas 4). After two treatments she began sleeping more easily and she was less tired. I asked her to do the Through-going Vessel stretching exercise at home. After three months her fatigue vanished and her cold hands and feet improved considerably. She became involved in her music once again.

DANCING SHOES

An attractive young woman, a classical dancer, consulted me about pain in her ankles, knees and lower back. When I examined her abdomen I found that her Spleen had a strong, rapid pulse and that her Liver was weak. The Yin and Yang Ankle Vessels and the Yin and Yang Linking Vessels were involved, something common in those who work with their body. The strong influence of the Yin Linking Vessel meridian implicated the Spleen, Heart Constrictor and Liver meridians.

Treatment This woman started out as a member of a very well-known company. When she became a freelance dancer, her discipline fell apart. She ate whatever came to hand and developed an intense craving for sweets. Then she started to notice pain in her ankles and knees, a joint pain that gradually climbed up to her back.

Young dancers often do not realize that what they eat has a direct influence on how they can express emotion through their bodies. I told this girl never to eat chocolate or sweets, and worked on her four times each day, stimulating the Yang and Yin Ankle Vessel meridians. I told her to do the Yin and Yang Ankle meridian stretching exercises. After four sessions, her joint pain disappeared. Because I persuaded her to stop eating snack foods and sweets, her concentration was soon restored.

MY ACHING BACK

An older woman came to see me because her lower back was in spasm and she could not walk. This was a chronic disorder. She went to an osteopath who would realign the vertebrae, but they would soon go out again. She was exhausted because of overwork and stress, and her nerves were fragile.

Treatment When I touched this woman's abdominal *Tanden* point, the great energy reservoir, I found it weak, empty and cold. I left my palm there for almost fifteen minutes until the area gradually warmed up. I worked on the lower part of the Kidney meridian. The right side was very rigid, so I applied enough pressure to release the tension. The next day she was considerably better; more than half of the pain was gone. The rest of the pain vanished in two treatments. Though it was impossible to work directly on her back, the leg meridians (Bladder, Kidney, Small Intestine and Liver) allowed me to put indirect pressure on the painful area.

Hands Up

A young man, a pianist, came to me with an arm problem. He literally could not raise his arm. The fifth and sixth thoracic vertebrae were so painful they could not be touched.

Treatment I realized the Small Intestine and the Heart meridians were involved in this problem. I worked on the fifth finger of each hand very carefully. I noticed the left finger, which corresponds to the Heart meridian, was deformed. I asked when the problem started and was told about six months previously. Thus the problem bordered on becoming chronic. I worked along the Governing Vessel meridian very gently to circulate yang energy. After four treatments he could move his arm, but the pain in the Heart region would return whenever he suffered emotional stress. It was a long time before the finger became fully supple again.

6

Shiatsu and the *I Ching*

The *I Ching* is a very old book of wisdom first used as an oracle, a way to understand the significance of what is happening to you in order to face a problem or challenge. Because it used what we now call yin and yang to create a picture of the moving world, the *I Ching* also became a treasury of medical and philosophical thought, collecting all the elements of time cycles, yin and yang theory and the theory of the Five Processes around its three-line and six-line divinatory diagrams (*gua*). As an oracle, it can help us understand the meaning of our problem. As a method of analysis, it can show us in precise detail how *ki* energy is moving through the body. As a way of thinking, it can orient us toward heaven and help us fight our compulsive and destructive egotism.

It is very important for us to understand the movement of energy in our body and to see how this connects us with the world around us. Just as the movements of air and water stabilize our planet, the exchange of hot and cold through the meridians stabilizes our body. A table made from the symbols of the *I Ching* shows this.

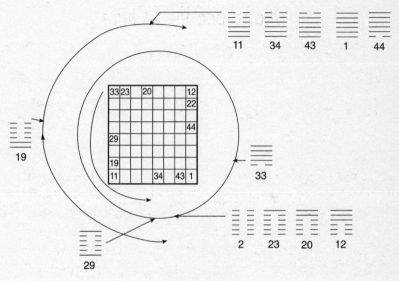

Circle of Life

The Outside Circle shows the movement of heaven or yang, while the Inside Square shows earth or yin. The small diagrams are *gua*, made up of solid (yang) and opened (yin) lines. Here they represent the twelve stages of the movement of yang energy, shown as a solid line, from beginning to extinction. Arranged in a line, these *gua* represent the tenuous balance that we walk along the border of life and death. We are totally dependent on nourishing the yang energy that connects us with heaven.

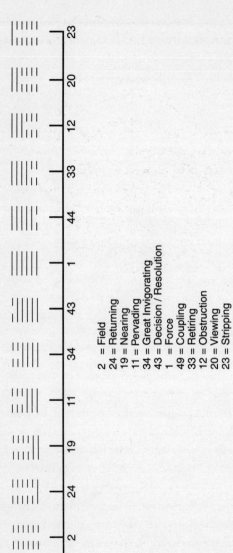

2 = Field
24 = Returning
19 = Nearing
11 = Pervading
34 = Great Invigorating
43 = Decision / Resolution
1 = Force
49 = Coupling
33 = Retiring
12 = Obstruction
20 = Viewing
23 = Stripping

Life Line

The square of earth also corresponds to the movement of the seasons and connects directly to our body.

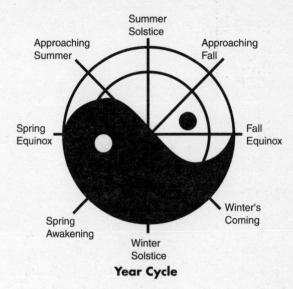

Year Cycle

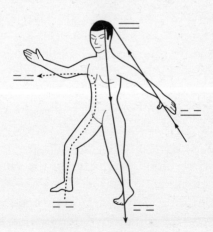

Seasons of the body

As in a year, there are also four seasons in our body, signified here by four sets of lines:

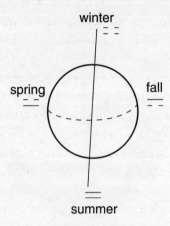

Season Lines

If we look at the diagram on page 207 we see that the circuits of the yang meridians in the body ascend, imitating the movement of heaven. They begin at the fingers, rise to a maximum, then drop toward the minimum. The yin meridians, beginning at the toes, enter into the depth of yin in the abdomen and chest, then continue to mount through the fingers. There is an exchange of heat and cold here, like the climate, but even more there is an exchange of *ki* energy (yang) and blood (yin). *Ki* is born in the yang areas, the hands and the head, while blood originates in the yin areas, feet and abdomen/chest.

The equilibrium between *ki* and blood is a central idea in oriental thought, connecting everything together: cosmology, medicine, philosophy and individual experience. Blood is a material element made up of various kinds of cells carried in plasma, but *ki* is an invisible element controlling its movement. This is the invisible power of heaven holding and controlling the material and concrete earth. We come from and return to the invisible, and we see this in every small part of ourselves.

The *I Ching* was first employed as an oracle. A medium (*wu*) prayed that the invisible force (*shen* or spirits) would descend to give us peace and happiness and drive away what is harmful. As time went on, however, we began to worship our own intellect in the place of the spirits. This is why the alarms have gone off, forcing us to realize that our earth, too, must be respected if it is to continue to support us all.

The Yellow Emperor's Classic of Internal Medicine, which in many ways is an extended commentary on the *I Ching*, is very explicit about this difference between *shen* as spirit and *shen* as ego-mind. The first is a global spirit of communication that presupposes we are all in the same boat. The second typifies someone who only thinks of their own interests to the detriment of others. Many of our institutions and businesses today are run by this greedy kind of 'thinking person'. But each of us can change at any point. I feel this is the great lesson of oriental 'wisdom' books, much more important than all of the very helpful techniques. Using Shiatsu, we can help the change in each person by dissolving what blocks the free circulation of energy and spirit.

YIN AND YANG IN THE PRINCIPAL MERIDIANS

We can also use the trigrams and hexagrams of the *I Ching* to look deeper into how the Principal Meridians work, and how they connect with the Extraordinary Meridians. The first step involves using the Eight Trigrams (*bagua*) of the *I Ching* to help us see how yin and yang play their part. Traditionally the Principal Meridians are arranged into six 'couples' or pairs by using the six 'mixed' trigrams that reflect the interplay of yin and yang. They become three yang couples and three yin couples, and the three-line diagrams from the *I Ching* show us what kind of yin or yang energy is at work in each pair, allowing a wide range of associations and correlations.

⚌ (trigram)	Tui
⚌ (trigram)	Sun
⚌ (trigram)	Li
⚌ (trigram)	Chen
⚌ (trigram)	Ken
⚌ (trigram)	K'an

Trigram Figures

The three yang couples are:

Bright Yang (*Yomei*), the trigram Lake (*Tui*)
Great Yang (*Taiyo*), the trigram Wind (*Sun*)
Small Yin (*Shiyo*), the trigram Fire (*Li*)

The three yin couples are:

Waning Yin (*Kechin*), the trigram Thunder (*Chen*)
Great Yin (*Taiyin*), the trigram Mountain (*Ken*)
Small Yang (*Shiyoyo*), the trigram Water (*K'an*)

Each couple is made up of two Principal Meridians:

Bright Yang:	Large Intestine Meridian
	Stomach Meridian
Great Yang:	Small Intestine Meridian
	Bladder Meridian
Small Yin:	Heart Meridian
	Kidney Meridian
Waning Yin:	Heart Constrictor Meridian
	Liver Meridian
Great Yin:	Lung Meridian
	Spleen-Pancreas Meridian
Small Yang:	Triple Warmer Meridian
	Gall Bladder Meridian

Thus we have six couples or pairs. As we can see in the following illustration, these couples of Principal Meridians are arranged around a special circle or eight-pointed compass shape. Two of the Extraordinary Meridians act as the vertical axis or pivot of this compass, the Governing Vessel and the Conception Vessel. The Governing Vessel meridian represents the zenith or highest point of yang energy, connected with the trigram Heaven (*Ch'ien*), while the Conception Vessel meridian represents the zenith of yin energy, represented by the trigram Earth (*K'un*). This is the Anterior Heaven Arrangement, or Arrangement According to Fu Hsi. All the Principal Meridian forces are symmetrically laid out, and ideally we can follow the movement of yin and yang through the meridians as they transform into each other.

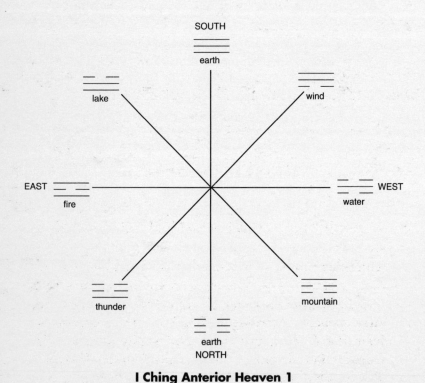

I Ching Anterior Heaven 1

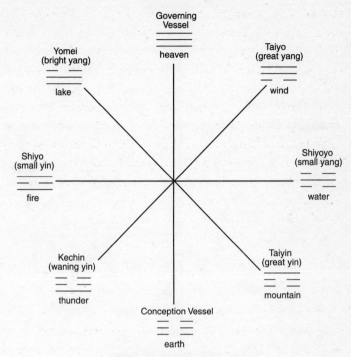

I Ching Anterior Heaven 2

ANOTHER HEAVEN, ANOTHER EARTH

This illustration shows another arrangement of the diagrams, the couples and their associations, an arrangement called the Posterior Heaven Arrangement or the Arrangement According to King Wen. This, too, comes from the *I Ching*, but much philosophy separates it from the first diagram. The first, the Anterior Heaven, shows what happens in an ideal or symmetrical

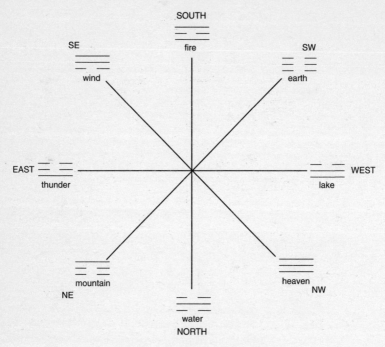

I Ching Posterior Heaven 1

world. The forces move back and forth in a balanced and understandable way. Here, in the Posterior Heaven, things have changed. The world has become much more complex. We encounter the forces of human society, and they are not always benign.

The *gua* or *I Ching* diagrams represent the basic forces and images we use to think about the world. The world itself is called Heaven and Earth (*t'ien ti*), a combination of the first two trigrams. Each of these eight three-line diagrams or trigrams represents a

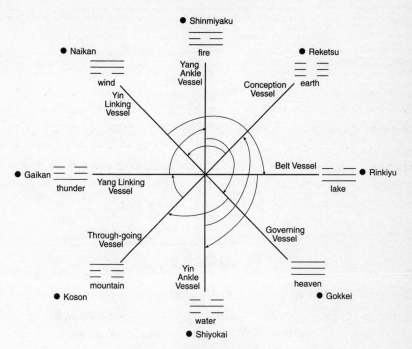

I Ching Posterior Heaven 2

spreading field of associations, fields that include the Principal Meridians. These fields of associations keep expanding; they are not dead categories, but live connections.

So the Eight Trigrams (*bagua*) represent many things. Here is a list of their basic associations. It is good to keep them in mind, and add to them through your own experience. This will tell you a lot about how the meridians work.

In the Posterior Heaven the diagrams are arranged

EIGHT TRIGRAMS AND THEIR ATTRIBUTES			
Trigram	Image	Action	Symbol
	Force Ch'ien	Persisting	Heaven
	Field K'un	Yielding	Earth
	Shake Chen	Stirring-up	Thunder
	Gorge K'an	Venturing Falling	Rushing water
	Bound Ken	Stopping	Mountain
	Ground Sun	Entering	Wood/Wind
	Radiance Li	Congregating	Fire Brightness
	Open Tui	Stimulating	Lake/Marsh

Trigram Table

in a very different way. Everything has been radically shifted. If we look at the illustrations, we can see how the Extraordinary Meridians fit into this picture. The key to this is number.

When we compare the position of the Eight Trigrams in the Anterior and Posterior Heaven Arrangements, we see that Heaven, Earth, and Lake have all moved three positions around the circle. Fire, Water, Wind and Mountain have all moved two places from their original positions, and thunder is one step from its original place.

If we look at the circle carefully we see that this movement has produced some very important changes. The sign for Earth has been placed *above* the sign for Heaven, indicating that these two powers are now *actively* connected, while the trigram for Lake is between them as mediator. This Lake sign, connecting the microcosm and the macrocosm, represents the Belt Vessel meridian. So just as Heaven and Earth interact, the Belt Vessel (one of the Extraordinary Meridians) co-ordinates the Conception Vessel (Yin Zenith) and the Governing Vessel (Yang Zenith). Through this we see that the Belt Vessel can provide us with a way to balance yin and yang energy in the events of our everyday lives and can adjust our practice accordingly.

Let us look further into these relations by using numbers, for they provide a clear illustration of the importance of the Extraordinary Meridians in the energy circulation of our bodies and lives. The Governing Vessel, the Conception Vessel, the Belt Vessel and the Through-going Vessel are the most important Extraordinary Meridians. Each of these, however, is coupled with another, similar, meridian: the Governing Vessel is coupled with the Yang Ankle Vessel (Heaven and Fire); the Conception Vessel is coupled with the Yin Ankle Vessel (Earth and Water); the Belt Vessel is coupled with the Yang Linking Vessel (Lake and Thunder); the Through-going Vessel is coupled with the Yin Linking Vessel (Mountain and Wind).

If we look at the steps around the circle these pairs have taken, we find something very interesting that reinforces our sense of the Extraordinary Meridians as transitional powers. Let us add them up. The Governing Vessel and the Yang Ankle Vessel together equal five (5). The Conception Vessel and the Yin Ankle Vessel together equal five (5). The Belt Vessel and the Yang Linking Vessel together equal four (4), and the

Through-going Vessel and the Yin Linking Vessel equal four (4). The total of these numbers is eighteen (18), an extremely important number for what we call *do yo*, the transition between the seasons. In Japanese reckoning, there are 18 days of transition between each season. Each season takes 72 days. There are four seasons (4 × 72 = 288) and four interseasonal earth elements (4 × 18 = 72). This earth element exists between each season, rather than being the end of summer we are familiar with. The Extraordinary Meridian can thus be seen as taking the place of the Earth element.

If we look at the Posterior Heaven Arrangement, we see that here the Extraordinary Meridians have taken the place of the Principal Meridians. Reflecting the complexity of living in our world, the Extraordinary Meridians connect things. They move back and forth, going in both directions around the circle. The lines and arrows drawn on this diagram show how these meridians work when we compare the positions with the Anterior Heaven Arrangement. This is a crucially important insight. The Extraordinary Meridians act to connect us with a more stable and more perfect state of being, something we can experience if our inner energies are in order.

Each of the Extraordinary Meridians has a regulating point that corresponds to one of the Five Processes or Elements. In oriental medicine, the Five Processes are a very important way to analyse energy movements. There are two basic cycles in Five Processes theory, a constructive cycle and a destructive cycle. In the constructive cycle, each process gives rise to another: wood creates

8 Extraordinary Vessels	Regulating Points	Five Elements
Governing Vessel	Gokkei - Small Intestine 3	Imperial fire
Conception Vessel	Reketsu - Lung meridian 7	Metal
Belt Vessel	Rinkiyu - Gall Bladder meridian 40	Wood
Through-going Vessel	Koson - Spleen-Pancreas meridian 4	Earth
Yang Ankle Vessel	Shinmiyaku - Bladder meridian 58	Water
Yin Ankle Vessel	Shiyokai - Kidney meridian 5	Water
Yang Linking Vessel	Gaikan - Triple Warmer meridian 5	Ministerial fire
Yin Linking Vessel	Naikan - Heart Constrictor meridian 6	Ministerial fire

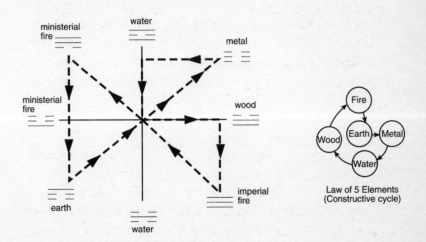

Law of 5 Elements
(Constructive cycle)

Process Cycles

fire, fire creates earth, earth creates metal, metal creates water, and water creates wood. To connect this with the Extraordinary Meridians, we divide the fire process into imperial fire and ministerial fire.

Again, if we look at these diagrams we see the great importance of the Extraordinary Meridians. Their job is above all to *connect* things throughout the world we live in and to provide a way for yin and yang energy to *circulate*.

USING *I CHING* TO ANALYSE YIN–YANG IMBALANCE

In eastern thought we also use the *I Ching* to understand the physiological aspects of yin and yang. Just like the natural world, our body has its directions: east, south, west and north. We visualize these directions by imagining a servant with his back facing north as he

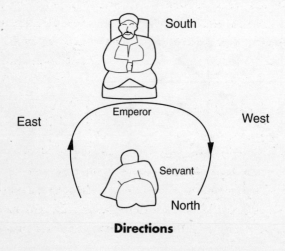

Directions

looks toward his lord in the south. (In the eastern compass, south is at the top.) His left side and arm will face east, his right side and arm will face west.

The east is sunrise and is associated with rising yang energy; the west is sunset and is associated with waning yang and the yin side of things. South is the zenith, the pinnacle of yang energy, while north is the most intense yin, the darkest and most obscure energy.

Once we determine left (east) and right (west), we can determine what is high or superior and what is low or inferior as indicators of the position of yin and yang in the body. High and low are defined by the navel or umbilical cord and the Belt Vessel, while left and right come from the Governing Vessel and the Conception Vessel. The Governing Vessel divides the back of the body into left and right, while the Conception Vessel divides the front of the body into left and right.

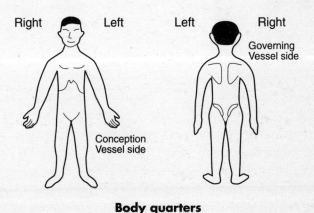

Body quarters

These three Extraordinary Meridians – Belt Vessel, Governing Vessel and Conception Vessel – make up the topological map of the yin–yang gradient in our body.

The Belt Vessel determines what is high and what is low. High is associated with yang and the south, low with yin and the north. It also connects the Conception Vessel (Point 8, *Shinketsu*, found between the second and third lumbar vertebrae) and the Governing Vessel (Point 4, *Meimon*), making a circle around the body.

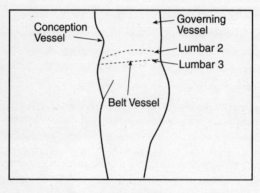

Belt vessel

If we look carefully at the Belt Vessel, we see that there are sixteen meridian points on the circle that it makes around the body. These sixteen meridian points represent the interconnections of sixteen hexagrams of the *I Ching*.

We can use these sixteen hexagrams to make eight topological maps of the yin–yang energies in our body. We start with the three-line diagrams or trigrams that

2	52	29	57	51	30	58	1
Field	Bound	Gorge	Penetrating	Shake	Radiance	Open	Force

11	41	63	42	32	64	31	12
Pervading	Diminishing	Already Fording	Augmenting	Persevering	Not Yet Fording	Conjoining	Obstruction

Hexagrams

make up the sixteen hexagrams. The posterior part of the body is associated with the yang family of trigrams: Heaven, Lake, Fire and Thunder. The most yang part of the body is the upper left side of the back associated with Heaven and the least yang part is the lower right side associated with Thunder. The front or anterior side of the body is associated with the yin family of trigrams: Wind, Water, Mountain and Earth. The most yin part of the body is the lower right front associated with Earth and the least yin part is the upper left front associated with Wind.

With the help of the *I Ching* hexagrams we can get a very clear picture of yin–yang balance and imbalance and how to diagnose and correct it. There are key points to use for each part of the body:

Left   Right   Right   Left

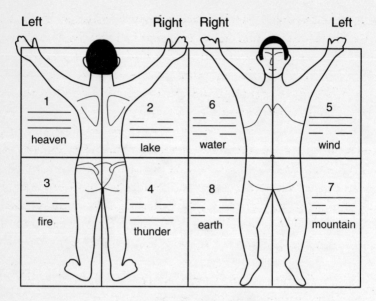

Front and back of body

- To diagnose and correct energy imbalance in the Heaven sphere, we look at two regulating points on the posterior side of the left arm: *Gokkei* (Small Intestine 3), the regulating point of the Governing Vessel, and *Gaikan* (Triple Warmer 5), the regulating point of the Yang Linking Vessel.

- To diagnose and correct energy imbalance in the Lake sphere, we look at the same two points on the posterior side of the right arm: *Gokkei* (Small Intestine 3), the regulating point of the Governing Vessel, and *Gaikan* (*Triple Warmer 5*), the regulating point of the Yang Linking Vessel.

- To diagnose and correct energy imbalance in the Fire sphere, we look at two regulating points on the left posterior side of the body: *Rinkiyu* (Gall Bladder 40), the regulating point of the Belt Vessel, and *Shinmiyaku* (Bladder 58), the regulating point of the Yang Ankle Vessel.

- To diagnose and correct energy imbalance in the Thunder sphere, we look at the same two regulating points on the right posterior side of the body: *Rinkiyu* (Gall Bladder 40), the regulating point of the Belt Vessel, and *Shinmiyaku* (Bladder 58), the regulating point of the Yang Ankle Vessel.

- To diagnose and correct energy imbalance in the Wind sphere, we look at two regulating points on the anterior side of the left arm: *Reketsu* (Lung 7), the regulating point of the Conception Vessel, and *Naikan* (Heart Constrictor 6), the regulating point of the Yin Linking Vessel.

- To diagnose and correct energy imbalance in the Water sphere, we look at the same two regulating points on the anterior side of the right arm: *Reketsu* (Lung 7), which is the regulating point of the Conception Vessel, and *Naikan* (Heart Constrictor 6), which is the regulating point of the Yin Linking Vessel.

- To diagnose and correct energy imbalance in the Mountain sphere, we look at two regulating points on the anterior lower left side of the body: *Koson* (Spleen-Pancreas 4), the regulating point of the Through-going Vessel, and *Shiyokai* (Kidney 5), the regulating point of the Yin Ankle Vessel.

• To diagnose and correct energy imbalance in the Earth sphere, we look at the same two regulating points on the anterior lower right side of the leg: *Koson* (Spleen-Pancreas 4), the regulating point of the Through-going Vessel, and *Shiyokai* (Kidney 5), the regulating point of the Yin Ankle Vessel.

In my experience, people who have serious chronic health problems tend to show an energy imbalance between the Heaven and Earth parts of the body. When the parts of the yin–yang combination are far apart they reflect a greater energy imbalance. For example, if we find blocked energy in Heaven's regulating points on the posterior side of the left arm (Small Intestine 3 and Triple Warmer 5), we will also find that the diagonal points on the other side of the body, Earth's regulating points, are also very blocked (Lung 7 and Heart Constrictor 6). More precisely, if the regulating points of Heaven are empty (*kyo*) the opposite points on the Earth side will be overcharged (*jitsu*), and the converse. The smaller the yin–yang difference, the milder the symptoms will be.

We can see these kinds of imbalance through four pairs of hexagrams from the *I Ching* and the Eight Trigrams (*bagua*) that compose them. Remember, the yang family of trigrams (Heaven, Lake, Fire and Thunder) represent the overcharged or *jitsu* condition, while the yin family (Earth, Mountain, Water, and Wind) represent the empty or *kyo* condition.

Hexagram combinations that indicate signs of significant imbalance are:

| 11 | 12 | 63 | 64 |
| Pervading | Obstruction | Already Fording | Not Yet Fording |

Hexagram combinations that indicate signs of lesser imbalance are:

| 41 | 31 | 42 | 32 |
| Diminishing | Conjoining | Augmenting | Persevering |

Combination	Symptoms
11 or 12	Chronic problems such as diabetes, neurological deficiency, hereditary problems, arthritis, rheumatism, high blood pressure, cancer, mental health problems, hysteria, nervous disorders, epilepsy.
31 or 41	Acute problems such as sciatica, lumbago, digestive problems, insomnia, allergies, sinusitis, problems with the large intestine.
63 or 64	Chronic problems including brain haemorrhage, heart disease, kidney stones, lack of energy, gynaecological problems.
32 or 42	Acute problems with digestive system, nervous system metabolism, muscular problems, weakness of liver, weakness of eyes.

A Table of Hexagram Pairs

- The greatest difference is represented by Hexagrams 11 and 12, Earth over Heaven and Heaven over Earth. In Hexagram 12, the upper regulating points are *jitsu* and the lower regulating points are *kyo*; in Hexagram 11 it is the reverse. The idea is the same in the other pairs, which represent decreasing levels of imbalance.

- In Hexagram 31 (Lake over Mountain), the upper points are *jitsu* or overcharged, while the lower points are *kyo* or empty; in Hexagram 41 (Mountain over Lake), the situation is reversed.

- In Hexagram 64 (Fire over Water), the upper points are *jitsu* or overcharged, while the lower points are *kyo* or empty; in Hexagram 63 (Water over Fire), the situation is reversed.

- The least amount of imbalance is represented by Hexagrams 32 and 42 (Thunder over Wind and Wind over Thunder). In Hexagram 32, the upper points are *jitsu* or overcharged and the lower are *kyo* or empty; in Hexagram 42, the reverse is true.

In my experience, when the yang or upper part of the hexagram is empty (11, 41, 63, 42) the energy imbalance is considerable greater than in those hexagrams where it is overcharged (12, 31, 64, 32).

Though there are many complex factors involved in the yin–yang balance of our bodies that a straightforward analysis may not answer, such a broad, clear picture can help us tremendously in our work. It is like the mathematical tool of a physicist or chemist who tries to apply his theoretical postulates to the infinitely complex natural world of the universe out there.

THE EXTRAORDINARY MERIDIANS AND HUMAN FORM

The diagrams and philosophy of *I Ching* can also help us to understand the evolution of the human form through the evolution of the meridians.

In the amoeba, one unified meridian enacts everything from within. The appearance of the fish shows the Governing Vessel appearing in the spine and the Conception Vessel in the abdomen. With reptiles, four limbs and the mobility that they represent appear. The next step, standing on two legs and liberating the arms to move freely in complex ways, gave us intelligence and sophistication in applying ourselves to survival.

In this context it is very important to note the crucial role the Gall Bladder meridian plays in the functioning of the Eight Extraordinary Meridians. It is directly connected to our human stance. It is represented by the Belt Vessel and plays a vital role in determining the eight differentiated yin–yang energy flows in our body. It is the only yang meridian that transports pure energy to the body, and is unique in that it touches all the other meridians as it pursues its path through our body. Simply standing up straight on two legs requires a con-

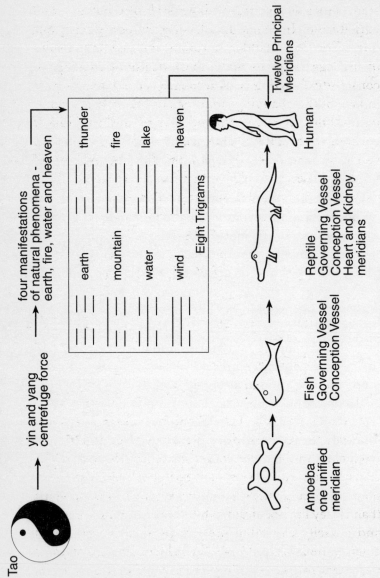

Tao

yin and yang
centrefuge force

four manifestations
of natural phenomena -
earth, fire, water and heaven

	earth			thunder
	mountain			fire
	water			lake
	wind			heaven

Eight Trigrams

Twelve Principal
Meridians

Amoeba
one unified
meridian

Fish
Governing Vessel
Conception Vessel

Reptile
Governing Vessel
Conception Vessel
Heart and Kidney
meridians

Human

Evolution

stant series of decisions about stability, balance and equilibrium. It demands a healthy response from our body. The Gall Bladder meridian, situated on the sides of the legs, helps us make these decisions to adapt to constantly changing circumstances, a real balancing act in face of the changing situations of life. It helps maintain stability in movement and thought in the middle of constant internal and external change. This constant active balance is the sign of a healthy body. The Gall Bladder meridian is also linked to the movement of the eyes, also crucial in maintaining balance.

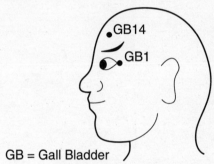

GB = Gall Bladder

Points for the eyes

According to *The Yellow Emperor's Classic of Internal Medicine*, the Gall Bladder meridian gives power and judgement to the eleven other Principal Meridians. For example, if people are afraid of getting sick through infection, they are actually much more likely to be infected than if they are not afraid, while those who show courage and tenacity can often prevent perverse energy from entering their body. The Gall Bladder meridian plays an important part in providing and sustaining this courage.

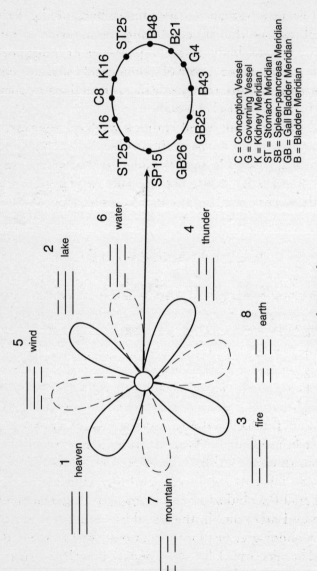

ST25
B48
B21
G4
K16 C8 K16
ST25
SP15
GB26 GB25 B43

C = Conception Vessel
G = Governing Vessel
K = Kidney Meridian
ST = Stomach Meridian
SB = Spleen-pancreas Meridian
GB = Gall Bladder Meridian
B = Bladder Meridian

2   6
lake   water

5
wind

4
thunder

8
earth

1
heaven

3
fire

7
mountain

Belt Vessel

If we now return to the illustrations of the Belt Vessel, we see that by combining the anterior or yin portions of the body with the posterior or yang portions, we can make a sort of geometrical diagram that represents the different yin–yang connections as they pass through the Belt Vessel.

All the yin–yang combinations we have seen pass through the Belt Vessel: Heaven to Earth, Lake to Mountain, Fire to Water, Thunder to Wind. Thus the Belt Vessel is the bridge of the yin and yang vessels and the exchange of energy that flows between them.

OUR BALANCING ACT

The Eight Extraordinary Meridians are constantly regulating the symmetrical balance between left and right, high and low, the surface and the depths of our body and the yin–yang energy that flows through it. This balancing act is vital to our existence as a biped, an animal that stands on two legs. Our stance has put our brain in the highest body position, creating intense brain stimulation as well as instability and the need to constantly adjust our balance. The main function of the Eight Extraordinary Meridians is to maintain this balance between left and right, high and low. Ever since the Industrial Revolution we have come to rely on machines more and more and in the last thirty years our use of new technologies has meant that our need to move or travel has decreased. The lack of use of our body causes it to degenerate. If we do not use our arms and legs, we create energy imbalance and internal stagnation arises, weakening our immune system and leaving us vulnerable to disease. So it is very important to do basic exercises that energize and balance our bodies. This is why the Eight Extraordinary Meridian stretching exercises are so important. In fifteen minutes per day we can maintain our basic balance and symmetry.

APPLYING THE SIXTY-FOUR HEXAGRAMS: THE HANDS OF FATE

In the east, we apply the sixty-four hexagrams of the *I Ching* to almost any kind of natural phenomena. Therapists often use the hexagrams to better understand our potential and our weaknesses. One method of doing this uses our fingerprints to examine both future potential and the impact of past events. To establish the hexagram combinations that let us examine these things, we must look at the fingers of both right and left hands.

There are three different kinds of patterns in our fingerprints. *Uzo*, the Spiral, represents a manifestation of Heaven; *Nagare*, Running Water, represents a manifestation of Earth; *Tomae*, Comma-shaped, represents a manifestation of the Human World. *Uzo* is represented by a yang line (———); *Nagare* and *Tomae* are represented by yin lines (— —). We can construct a hexagram from these lines, and use it to determine a wide range of associations. We usually draw an age line between past and future at about

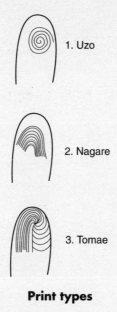

Print types

thirty-six years old for both men and women. Events
before that age are read on the right hand; events
after that age are read on the left. We read from the
little finger to the thumb, assigning a yin or yang line
to each finger.

For example, in the case of someone over thirty-six
years of age suppose the little finger on someone's left
hand is a Spiral sign (*Uzo*), as is the ring finger. Both
would be yang lines. The middle finger is a Running
Water (*Nagare*) sign, which is a yin line. But the middle
finger always takes two lines, for there are six lines to a
hexagram and only five fingers; so, as the centre of anything is considered to be very important in Chinese
thought, this would be a double yin line. The index

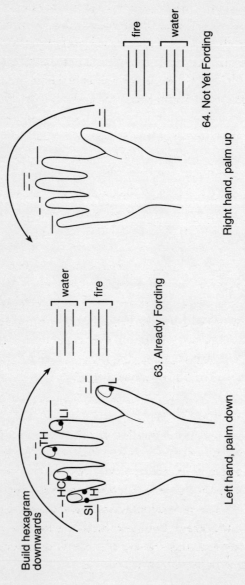

Build hexagram downwards

HC
TH
LI
SI
H
L

]water
]fire

63. Already Fording

Left hand, palm down

]fire
]water

64. Not Yet Fording

Right hand, palm up

Hand lines and hexagrams

finger of this person's hand is Comma-shaped (*Tomae*) and is thus a yin line, and the thumbprint is a Spiral (*Uzo*), which is a yang line. By putting these lines together from the bottom up, we get a hexagram, in this case No. 41. The lower trigram is Lake and the upper trigram is Mountain.

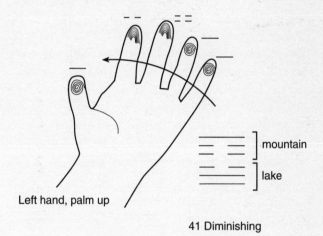

Left hand, palm up

] mountain

] lake

41 Diminishing

Hand lines and hexagrams

Next we determine which lines correspond to which parts of the body. Further, each of the trigrams has a strong point or central focus. The tables below give these correspondences. This strong point means the corresponding body part is vulnerable; in the case of Hexagram 41, with the trigrams Lake and Mountain, the vulnerable areas are the third line, which corresponds to the hip, and the sixth line, which corresponds to the neck and head.

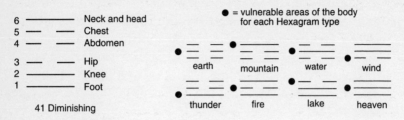

6 ———————— Neck and head
5 —— —— Chest
4 —— —— Abdomen

3 —— —— Hip
2 ———————— Knee
1 ———————— Foot

41 Diminishing

● = vulnerable areas of the body
   for each Hexagram type

earth   mountain   water   wind

thunder   fire   lake   heaven

Body Table

There is also a set of correspondences to the months of the year, so we can further say that the vulnerable times for this person (third and sixth line) are March, June, September and December.

June + Dec ——————— 6
May + Nov —— —— 5
Apr + Oct —— —— 4
Mar + Sept —— —— 3
Feb + Aug ——————— 2
Jan + July ——————— 1
41 Diminishing

Month Table

To find organ correspondences we use the connection of the Five Processes and the Eight Trigrams. In the case of Hexagram 41, the Mountain trigram corresponds with earth and the Lake trigram with metal, giving us an earth–metal relation. Earth corresponds to the Spleen and the Pancreas, while metal corresponds to the Lungs. In terms of the relation of the Five Processes, earth enhances metal, so we can say that the Spleen function activates the Lung function in a constructive way. Here is a table of the Five Processes and their connections to the Trigrams and the Organs.

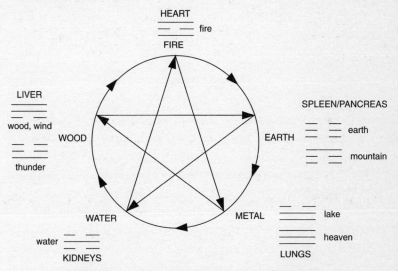

Five Processes with Trigrams and Organs

This hexagram can also give us an image of the innate character of the person through what is called the Nuclear Diagram. In the case of Hexagram 41, if we take lines 2, 3 and 4 as the lower trigram (Thunder) and lines 3, 4 and 5 as the upper trigram (Earth) we have the Hexagram 24, which means the return of yang energy. Here the vulnerable areas are lines 1 and 5, which correspond to the foot and chest, the earth process Spleen-Pancreas and the wood process Liver.

The Five Agent relationship here is the opposite of

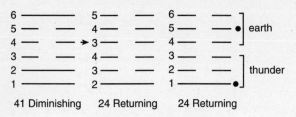

Nuclear Hexagram

41: the wood agent corresponding to the Liver attacks the earth process of the Spleen-Pancreas. This is the Destructive Cycle of the Five Processes, where wood covers earth. These Nuclear Hexagrams are used primarily to diagnose congenital or hereditary problems, problems that repeat generation after generation.

The primary hexagram that describes this person, No. 41, is called Diminishing. The image is the water of the Lake evaporating to enrich the vegetation of the Mountain, but the same water that enriches Heaven's Mountain will return to the Lake in the end as rain. A person with this sign on their hand will probably be very generous without knowing how to calculate the cost. They would not be good in business or commerce, and would be more likely to be a religious person or a teacher. This is the sign of altruistic people. This person is not afraid of exposing him or herself to danger for the sake of helping others.

Here is another example: a person whose right hand has the little finger pattern *Tomae* (Comma), which is a yin line; the ring finger *Uzo* (Spiral), which is a yang

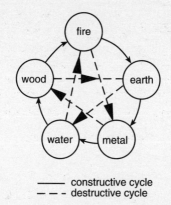

—— constructive cycle
– – – destructive cycle

Destructive and Constructive Cycles

line; the middle finger *Uzo* (Spiral), which gives two yang lines; the index finger *Nagare* (Running Water), which is a yin line; and the thumb *Nagare* (Spiral), another yin line. If we combine these lines, from bottom to top, we get Hexagram 32, which is called Persevering.

This hexagram is made up of Wind and Thunder and thus has vulnerable areas at the first and fourth lines, which represent the foot and the abdomen and the months of January, April, July and October. Both Thunder and Wind are wood, corresponding to the Liver. Whenever a process is doubled like this it indicates a great vulnerability or weakness in the organ involved. This doubled wood element reinforces the vulnerability of the Liver. This weakness of the first and fourth lines can be interpreted as a Liver weakness in the abdomen and in the Achilles tendon of the foot. The person who has this sign will have a hot temper and get angry quickly. He or she makes both friends and enemies easily. Such a person will have many new ideas but be unable to stick with them. This is an inventor who likes to create things but is never able to perfect them.

7

Shiatsu Workshop

With some understanding now of general Shiatsu, let us look at a typical workshop. It may help you to feel the interconnection of techniques, sensitivity, philosophy and pragmatism a new Shiatsu practitioner should learn. This workshop occurred several years ago when my father was still alive.

This workshop was held in an Italian seaside resort for about thirty people, who lived and worked together for a week. Many of them had become interested in Shiatsu through their work as masseurs and beauticians and had already acquired the fundamentals. This was an intensive course in theory and practice and centred on demonstrations and pair work through which people could have first-hand experience of the various techniques. A special atmosphere of caring and compassion develops in such a workshop in which the learning is shared by all.

My father and I were very interested in making the fundamentals of Shiatsu available in the west, and we would often teach together. The workshop was also an opportunity for us to explore the healing techniques and problems we were most interested in. It gave the participants a chance to experience a really remarkable combination of theory and practice in a very special atmosphere.

I deeply admired my father's strength, flexibility, sensitivity and intuition. He worked with both thumbs and toes, using a series of wooden rods capped with silver that allowed him to apply pressure at precise angles to different parts of the body. It was like trapping a bird or watching a burglar to see that quality of stealth and precision.

My father was interested in the brain. I wanted him to be able to work with brain specialists and neurologists. What does medicine feel about the brain? Does the skull breathe? Can the brain absorb blood (yin) from outside? The brain controls exercise, and the brain gets tired, using enormous amounts of oxygen and nutrients. The fatigue people feel through brainwork comes from the blood as it starts to coagulate.

My father was also very interested in stomach problems and the vagus nerve, which connects the brain and the stomach. Take the eyeball, for example, a delicate piece of anatomy that lies very close to the brain. Control the blood supply there, he said, and you control the blood flow to the brain.

We practised Zen Shiatsu, which talks a lot about the

lymph system and how it is overlooked in Western medicine. The neglect is in direct proportion to attention given to the brain. My father worked by sensing this neglect. His thumbs were like dowsing tools detecting the blocked energy. The head and the brain are the first parts of the body to deteriorate, dramatically so after the age of fifty. That is why my father worked so much on his own head. The spine and the circulation of the blood are crucially important to a feeling of well being.

Eat regularly! Father had breakfast and lunch at 11.30, went to the toilet precisely at 2.30, had supper at 7.30 and went to bed at midnight. He always reclined after meals to aid digestion. He felt that natural foods were important. Natural sugar tastes a bit sour, while artificial sugar erodes the arteries and absorbs calcium. Cigarettes are *very bad*!

So many of my patients have said, 'I wish you could give me a treatment to help me simply stop smoking and drinking too much.' This is everyone's dream. But my father had the *will* to do it. After meals he went into the state of being empty we call *mogano koji*, and he practised *messemso*, one-point concentration, like a samurai. He used it in Shiatsu to attack the patient's problem.

FIRST DAY

It was almost dark when the boat landed at Ishia, pitch black when we got to the hotel. The sea was pounding against the rocks, lashed on by the rain and wind, and it became more and more of a presence at dinner. Sitting with the organizers of the seminar at the head table, I said, 'The sea on one side, mountains on the other and the hot mineral baths in front – what more could you want?'

After dinner I gave a treatment to a particular friend who was one of the participants. 'Your back is bad now,' I said. I walked on her feet, after probing with my thumbs down a double column on both sides of her spine. I couldn't break through her congested breathing. I finished by stroking her head. It felt like a mossy tree trunk.

SECOND DAY

This morning I gave a demonstration of technique and a lesson about how our bodies are made. We worked in pairs. Each person would run the heel of their hand down their partner's back, left of centre with the right hand, three times, then right of centre with the left hand, three times. Then they would follow the same path with their thumbs, five fingers below the ribs, three times, then behind the head, then four points that outline the scapula.

The participants took notes and practised in pairs. The room was full of wicker mats and three-foot-long blue sausage pillows. It looked out on the mineral pools which were burrowed into the hill. Outside was a sun terrace, with stacks and stacks of wooden chairs.

SECOND DEMONSTRATION

After lunch on Sunday I felt we needed to experience how the skin and the lungs were connected. The yang meridian here is the Triple Warmer and the yin meridian is the Heart Ruler. I drew them in a circle, the cycle of the Five Processes: fire and the heart are the circulatory system at the top; earth is Digestion at the centre of the circle; metal is the Respiratory System on the right hand; water eliminates and regenerates below; wood is Digestion, which covers earth, Muscles and Liver. It stands on the left at the point of the new spring. We can see this cycle two ways: as a circle it is a restorative cycle, as a star is destructive.

I also instructed the women in using Shiatsu to deal with menstrual disorders. In the sitting position (*badakonasana*) they stroke the tibia, where the very important Spleen-Pancreas meridian drops down from the knee. Stroke this spot and follow the meridian down with your thumb three times each day. Then rotate the big toes quickly and firmly, and press the Liver meridian points inside the big toe.

We took a swim after the long day. The water was very hot on the surface, but cool a few inches down. Everyone went into the water. Playing.

THIRD DAY

I drew a diagram that connected points along the spine with all the major disorders, almond-shaped patterns down the back, starting below the inverted triangles of the scapulae.

Meridian	Element	Problem
Lungs	Metal	psychological, circulation
Heart/	Fire	deep circulation problems
Heart Ruler		and psychological blocks; collects bad energy
Pancreas	Earth	digestive problems
Intestine	Fire	assimilation and retention
Kidney	Water	elimination, sex, urogenital

Fire rises, earth is at the centre, water sinks. Metal is not heavy because it receives cosmic energy. The Pancreas is the meeting ground and transformational centre of the two energies. It defends and nourishes, while the Heart circulates the energy.

All work should come from the centre, the deep abdomen breathing that unites metal and fire. The Japanese word *semei* shows this. It combines birth and individuality with fate. Our deep centre does not separate past or future from the present. We are all part of the great 'collective unconscious'.

FOURTH DAY

Today we began with stretches, first individually, then in pairs. We walked on each other's thighs, sitting on our heels, lying back with our arms over our heads.

We then moved into thumb pressure along the Bladder meridian, deep pressure, slow exhaling from the *hara* (low abdomen) following the fifth to tenth points. We did this three times, with the fingers always in contact. Then we worked around the sacrum and along the line of four points that joined the hip and leg on the outside of the body. This was almost always painful. We slid the heel of the hand along the outside of the thigh, along the Gall Bladder meridian. The hands are always yin and yang. The yang hand is the working hand; the yin hand is the stabilizing hand.

We ended with another discussion of the Five Processes, keyed to the seasons. Fire above is summer, Blood and the bitter taste. Earth at the centre is late summer. Metal at the right is autumn, the Lungs and the colour white. Water below is winter, the Kidneys and the colour black. Wood on the left is spring and the Liver.

Two important terms emerged from this discussion. *Jitsu* means too much energy, and is usually the effect. *Kyo* means too little energy, and is usually the cause.

FIFTH DAY

Today I concentrated on the cranium. The Animation Point, located at the top of the head between the ears, is one of the most important points in Shiatsu. It is called *Hiyakue* in Japanese, and lies on the Governing Vessel meridian. First we worked on all the Governing Vessel points on the top of the head, using our thumbs one on top of the other, our fingers spread out to the sides like a butterfly's wings. The butterfly's wings are the symbol of Shiatsu.

There are two rows of five points in front of *Hiyakue*, and three rows of five points behind it. We worked from front to back along the centre rows, and from back to front along the outside rows, then we applied deep pressure to the *Hiyakue* point three times. The treatment ended with deep pressure three times on the two points just in front of the *Hiyakue* point. Throughout this treatment, the right hand applies pressure and the left holds it firm. You finish by vibrating your palms on the temples, hands over the eyes and elbows stiff.

On the front of the body there are five rows of seven points spaced across the chest, centred on the sternum. The Conception Vessel meridian goes up the centre of this field. This is where emotional blockage can be released. The fifth point down from the clavicle is very important for the heart and emotional life. Working from side to side along all these points benefits the lungs.

TREATMENT

I gave a second treatment to my friend who was participating in the workshop. As she lay on her stomach, I put deep pressure on all the points that lay along the spine, then walked on her feet. As she lay on her back, I probed the points around the solar plexus. I worked on the head points that felt so far away yesterday, asking 'How does it feel here? How does this famous point feel?'

All of these points were much closer to the surface.

Yesterday they were mossy, the days before low, stiff and sore. They were sensitive now. This would awaken lots of memories.

THINKING OF HEAVEN

Heaven energy enters through the *Hiyakue* point and plunges down to the *Tanden* point in the abdomen. Heaven energy also enters through the nose with an in breath and travels down to the *Tanden* point. This is the energy that works, subtle and sensitive. It is recharged in the *Tanden* and freed by exhaling through the mouth. The *Yusen* point in the foot, just under the Conception point, is the entry for earth energy. Flexible shoes and contact with the ground can draw this energy and capture it. That is why wood and straw are used for footwear in Japan.

DIAGNOSIS

Oriental diagnosis is made in four ways:

- *Boshin*: studying a person's appearance, the shape of their face, their colour and characteristic movements.
- *Bunshin*: listening to the voice, their sounds and odours.
- *Monshin*: conducting a dialogue, using indirect questions and psychological probing.
- *Setsushin*: direct touch and contact.

For Shiatsu, the most important method is Setsushin or direct touch. I gave everyone an example, working with the woman in class who had swollen bunions. With what we had already studied, we could predict the scar that showed she had had bronchial tube surgery and knew she was taking heavy doses of antibiotics.

TIME AND ENERGY

Each of the meridians is associated with a certain time of day. The meridians themselves come in threes or triangles. Where their points meet they create an opposition, and where their broad bases meet, they create harmony and conciliation.

Meridian	Energy	Time
Lungs	yin	3.00–5.00
Large Intestine	yang	5.00–7.00
Stomach	yang	7.00–9.00
Spleen	yin	9.00–11.00
Heart	yin	11.00 –13.00
Small Intestine	yang	13.00–15.00
Bladder	yang	15.00–17.00
Kidneys	yin	17.00–19.00
Heart Constrictor	yin	19.00–21.00
Triple Warmer	yang	21.00–23.00
Gall Bladder	yang	23.00–1.00
Liver	yin	1.00–3.00

Further, desire for a specific object creates a deficiency or lack in the Heart. When we try to reach out to this object of desire, it creates a block or rigidity in the Gall Bladder and the Liver. Meditation restores us to our centre and frees us from the desires.

'What about this little toe?' my patient asked. It was rudimentary; the nail had vanished and the tip was overgrown with forests of callus.

'Bladder and Kidneys,' I said, 'and ancestral energy. Stress draws on these reserves. And it shows great resistances.'

PARTNER WORK

We did abdominal analysis in pairs. This is a subtle form of diagnosis, and I did not expect people to master it at the first go. One pair could not find anything. The first partner told me her 'friend' must be perfectly healthy. I knelt at her right side and probed into her stomach. There was resistance at several points low in the abdomen. Her liver was overworked and her kidneys were weak.

If you are using this kind of diagnosis, you must first probe on the surface and only gradually deepen your exploration. Work the major points three times with the heel of the hand, then three times with three fingers of the right hand, then finally three times using the thumb or crossed thumbs. Work in a circle around the navel, pressing on eight different points. To finish, use waving motions and rolling motions across the abdomen and gently shake the low back in the region of the kidneys.

LAST DAY

We worked with the special, vital meridians, the Heart Constrictor or Heart Ruler meridian and the Triple Warmer meridian. Heaven energy enters at the top of the head and through the nose as we inhale and settles in the abdomen. Earth energy enters through the feet and through the mouth, through eating. It, too, goes to the abdomen. The Triple Warmer deals with the three functions of this energy.

Think of the body as divided in three parts. The first part, above the diaphragm, includes the Heart and Lungs. Here the Triple Warmer produces *superior* energy. The middle section of the body, including the Spleen, Liver and Pancreas, is where the Triple Warmer controls the production of *defensive* energy. Below the belt are the Kidneys, where hereditary and ancestral forces are at work and the Triple Warmer produces *sexual* energy.

Seishin is a Japanese word that means soul and individual spirit. These are the gift of the Way or *Tao*, the great vision of the world that is not earned but offered. The Heart and the Heart Ruling Vessel guard this energy as the pericardium guards the heart. Defensive energy, produced in the mid-section, is superficial. Nutritive energy, product of the deep abdomen, is more profound. The Governing Vessel and the Conception

Vessel control the flow of *seishin*. All emotional and psychological problems are manifested and controlled through the Heart Ruler meridian. The Heart, Lungs, Liver and Kidneys are the most important sources of these disturbances.

ENDING SONG

As we ended our Shiatsu session, we all learned and sang this old Japanese song:

> *Shiatsu no*
> Shiatsu is like
> *Koko ro ha ha*
> The waves in the sea.
> *Go ko ru o se ba*
> When they shove on like the wind,
> *Lino chino i zum*
> The waves one reaches
> *Waku ha ha ha*
> (Are like) the springs of (our) lives.

8

Treating Specific Disorders

Traditional oriental medicine deals with the whole individual, not just with symptoms, but it is sometimes necessary to focus on specific problems and diseases. Here Shiatsu techniques can come to your aid, helping you deal with your own situation so that you do not need to visit the doctor so often. Sickness often has a purpose, making you aware of the need for change. You can question your symptoms and seek their purpose and meaning. As you see into your condition, the problem will often solve itself and the flow of life move on.

These suggestions for treatment are aimed mainly at those who have acquired a basic working knowledge of Shiatsu techniques. There are now many groups and individuals teaching Shiatsu in most western countries. If you are interested in using these techniques, I would strongly recommend taking an introductory course with a recognized practitioner in your area. This is how the tradition is really passed on, through direct experience.

ANOREXIA AND BULIMIA

The anorexic refuses to eat, while the bulimic abnormally wants to eat everything put in front of them. Both show serious psychological and emotional imbalance. Many anorexics have gone through a terrible, tortuous relationship and their refusal of food is a refusal of this burden, a refusal to sustain life. Many bulimics have no deep love relationship they can trust and are full of long-term, pent-up frustration. They eat without ceasing to fill their emotional emptiness.

Treatment There are many degrees of these disorders. Some, characterized by serious pathological symptoms, require immediate psychological care. Others, which are characterized by periodic lapses, benefit greatly from the Governing Vessel stretching exercise and the Yin Linking Vessel stretching exercise. Work on all the meridians on the head, especially the path of the Governing Vessel, will be of benefit.

One of the most important aspects of Shiatsu treatment is that it works with the hands, like a painter or pianist. In addition to specific therapy, through our hands we can directly offer warmth, encouragement and care to these people who so desperately need it.

ASTHMA

This word comes from the Greek word for *panting*. The symptoms include spasmodic contraction of the bronchi, which impedes breathing. Asthma can be an allergic reaction or a psychological response to the environment, and it may be genetic. Contrary to common belief, people with asthma find it more difficult to exhale fully that to inhale.

Asthma is usually not life-threatening, but it can be extremely distressing. If it becomes chronic and is medicated with cortisone, there may be severe side-effects. Each asthma attack becomes more severe, needing urgent hospital attention. Many people suffer asthma attacks just before dawn, a time the clock of the meridians assigns to lung circulation.

Treatment Before treating this condition it is important to wait until the asthma attack has subsided. Find out if the patient is taking medication, for Shiatsu can provoke a serious negative reaction. People with chronic asthma tend to have weak Kidney and Spleen-Pancreas meridians and thus they prefer foods with pronounced tastes, sweet, spicy or salty, as well as strong coffee or tea.

Work on the Conception Vessel and its Regulator Point (*Reketsu*), linking it with the Lung meridian. In chronic cases, the Kidney Source Point and the Source Point of the Spleen-Pancreas meridian (*Taihaku*) will be empty. Work on the Conception and Through-going Vessels. When you examine the spinal column, which is linked with the Governing Vessel, you will often find the second and third thoracic vertebrae markedly concave and painful if pressed. This pain may also be felt around the fifth, sixth or seventh thoracic vertebrae. The Spleen and Kidney meridians are both important here in energizing the immune system. Allergy and asthma are a deterioration of the immune system facing the attack of chemicals, animal fats and environmental pollution.

Interestingly, people who have this problem are often perfectionists. They often suffer from migraine, another complaint common among those who insist on doing everything right. They may have asthma during one stage of their life and later develop eczema.

Both asthma and eczema are linked with the functioning of the Lung meridian. Preventative measures are easy. Eat a balanced diet, avoid rich foods and do the Conception and Through-going Vessel stretching exercises. If the exercises are too hard, press the regulator points of these vessels first.

CANCER

This is one of the last diseases to hold out against modern medicine. Shiatsu cannot cure cancer, but it can assist the body's natural resistance. The aim of treatment is not to do away with the symptoms, but to preserve what health is left. Once a disease has reached a pathological level, it becomes a medical problem and should be handled by doctors and hospitals. We can, however, offer considerable help in combating the side effects of radical medical treatments, such as weakness, vomiting, lack of appetite, depression and insomnia.

The Chinese ideogram for cancer is *gan*. It shows a person lying on a bed and three hard stones. Cancer is a hard, stone-like disease. The Japanese word suggests inflexibility, having a rigid head and a general lack of resilience. People who get cancer often have obstinate, inflexible thoughts. Once they decide on something, nothing stops them.

Visiting a religious shrine, I saw cancer patients miraculously cure themselves. These people had come together for a month to rekindle their sense of the spirit, to learn how to appreciate a simple existence and show gratitude to their parents and ancestors. This had nothing to do with modern medicine. It is a reminder that, if the conditions are right, we all have the hidden power to transform ourselves. Cancer comes from within, when healthy cells suddenly become malignant. It can be cured from within by a deep change of heart.

CIRCULATION PROBLEMS

Such conditions in the extremities or in the lower back are particularly common among women. Anaemia, hormonal imbalance and a malfunctioning autonomic nervous system are the most frequent causes. Oriental medicine looks at this problem in terms of overabundant *ki* energy and insufficient blood. Blood is the main supplier of nourishment to many parts of the body. Because women lose blood during their menstrual cycle, there is always a lack of blood in proportion to *ki*.

Treatment People who suffer from cold extremities and poor circulation benefit from exercising the Conception, Through-going and Governing Vessels. However women should avoid Conception Vessel exercises during their menstrual period. They can concentrate on exercising the Governing Vessel and the Through-going Vessel coupled with deep breathing.

CIRRHOSIS

This is the most serious liver problem. There are three types: one occurs when a massive number of liver cells die; another develops out of chronic hepatitis, resulting in blocked blood flow to the liver; the third is a direct result of excessive drinking. Normal liver function can often be re-established when the patient stops drinking.

Cirrhosis is usually detected only in its advanced stages. Symptoms include a feeling of being very full, constipation, loss of appetite and nausea. In advanced cases, the patient may vomit blood or have blood in his stool.

Treatment Shiatsu treatment is particularly beneficial before the symptoms are too advanced for it helps maintain balanced circulation. The Belt Vessel and the Yang Ankle Vessel are very helpful. In an advanced condition, the patient cannot do any of the exercises and treatment must be very gentle. Sometimes a gentle touch on the meridians is enough. Good food and a balanced life are a crucial part of the recovery process. Avoid stress and adopt a balanced diet that includes organically grown vegetables. Avoid frozen foods, carbonized water, sugar and alcohol.

CYSTITIS

This bladder inflammation is caused by intestinal bacteria or exposure to humid cold. Characteristic symptoms are pain in the urethra after urination, a feeling of urine remaining in the bladder and the frequent wish to urinate.

Treatment The patient should keep warm and avoid cold drinks. Work on the Conception Vessel and the Yang Ankle Vessel. The Bladder meridian in the leg, particularly Point 36 (*Ichu*) and the Bladder Source Point 60 (*Keikotsu*) will be very sensitive. Stretch these meridians after the acute symptoms have eased.

DEPRESSION

This word comes from a Latin word that means *down*. It is a common problem and has a variety of causes. In acute cases, it can interfere with sleep and lead to excessive drinking or suicide.

Depression is more common in northern climates where darkness can bring emotional lows. Often people suffering from depression are afraid to look at themselves in a mirror. If the mind is not correctly guided, it can cut the self and the body into small pieces, constructing an isolated, small being completely disconnected from the real world.

Treatment Shiatsu can be a very real help in depression. Work particularly on the Governing Vessel and the Yang Ankle Vessel and the exercises connected with them.

DIABETES MELLITUS

This is a metabolic disorder. When the pancreas functions normally, it secretes enough insulin to regulate the metabolism of carbohydrates, amino acids and fats. A malfunctioning pancreas leads to hyperglycaemia, too much sugar in the blood, and polyuria, too much glucose in the urine. Symptoms include thirst, hunger, physical weakness and emaciation, which can lead to a coma. Diabetes particularly occurs in industrialized countries. It is called the rich man's disease because it is associated with a high-calorie diet. The oriental approach to this problem is to modify the diet and increase the amount of exercise.

Treatment Work on the Spleen-Pancreas, the Through-going and the Yin Linking Vessel meridians helps, but the problem is usually quite deep-seated. After a prolonged period of weakness, the Spleen-Pancreas meridian will actually weaken the Kidneys and the body's immune system. The regulator point of the Through-going Vessel will be painful and cold to the touch. Stimulate this point, then work on the meridian itself. Though diabetes is directly caused by a lack of insulin, it is important to strengthen the overall balance of the hormonal system, for it is the hormonal system that co-ordinates muscles, tissues and organs.

DIZZINESS

This often bothers women in the early stages of pregnancy, while ear problems and low blood pressure are also accompanied by dizziness. With advancing age, difficult exercises must be avoided, but you can always apply pressure to the important points.

Treatment Press the Heart Constrictor Point 6 (*Naikan*) and the Triple Warmer Point 5 (*Gaikan*) ten to twenty times per day. This daily pressure is particularly useful for people with low blood pressure.

ECZEMA

This word comes from the Greek *ekzcin*, meaning to boil out. The condition, most often found in babies and children, is a superficial inflammation that makes the skin red and itchy. It most often appears on the face or the joints of the arms or legs, but may be found anywhere on the body. Eczema is connected with the Lung and Spleen-Pancreas meridians, especially the wet, humid type of eczema. It can be provoked by allergies to cow's milk, animal fur or certain food additives, as well as excessive acidity in the system. Children's eczema often reflects difficulties in the parents' relationship. When the difficulties are resolved, the eczema often disappears.

Treatment Work on the Through-going Vessel and the Yin Linking Vessel. Encourage reflection on the psychological sources of the disorder.

FEVERS

Shiatsu treatments should never be given to anyone with fever or high blood pressure. Wait until the acute symptoms subside to work on the meridians. Shiatsu stimulates the body's natural healing power and works with the natural processes of time and fever is part of this healing process. The body is trying to burn off accumulated toxins and kill the invading bacteria or virus. During a fever, the body's energy is concentrated on directly combating the problem. Shiatsu applied at the wrong time can divert this energy away from its proper focus.

A fever can also obscure other serious problems. A fever combined with a severe headache can indicate meningitis; a fever combined with an earache can indicate a serious infection of the inner ear. Jaundice, also characterized by a high fever, afflicts the Liver and Gall Bladder, and rheumatism can bring on a fever accompanied by pain in the lumbar region and aching joints. These are serious problems. They signal you to consult a doctor at once. Once the fever has subsided, however, you can begin to work.

Treatment Start with the forearm points on the Lung meridian, concentrating on the Arm Joint Point *Shiyakutaku* (Lung Point 5). Normally, after a fever this point will be painful to the touch. Work on the Triple Warmer meridian of the forearm and, before going to sleep, do the Governing Vessel meridian stretch. When you begin to sneeze, a sign that marks the onset of a fever, avoid cold drinks. Drink warm or hot drinks and keep your abdomen warm. Avoid alcohol. Eat very lightly or not at all.

GASTROPTOSIS

This is a Greek word for a 'slipped stomach' that has fallen below its normal position. It is characterized by gurgling sounds because of liquids retained in the stomach. This is a *kyo* or 'empty of energy' phenomenon. When an organ lacks energy it cannot maintain its proper position. This energy is normally supplied by the Stomach and Spleen-Pancreas meridians, which have abundant supplies of blood (*ketsu*) and *ki* energy.

Treatment Work on the Stomach meridian. Focus on the abdomen and legs. In chronic cases, look at the feet and toes. The feet are linked with Little Yang (*Shiyoyo*), which is yang in yin and belongs to the yin family. It has a very close connection to the internal organs. You can diagnose stomach problems by examining the second toe. The Stomach meridian terminates here, then connects with the Spleen-Pancreas meridian in the big toe. There is often a gap between them, as if energy were escaping. In a young child, these toes are close together, and the Buddha, too, is depicted with perfect feet. To treat the condition indicated by these signs, work on the Through-going Vessel. The partner exercises described earlier are also very beneficial.

GOUT

This comes from the Latin *gutta*, which means *a drop*. It was an ancient belief that this disease was caused by the slow dripping of a noxious liquid on to the inflamed joint. Gout is caused by excessive uric acid in the bloodstream. Like diabetes, those who suffer from gout overindulge in rich food and drink. Gout can be excruciatingly painful; the big toe can become so swollen that it is impossible to walk and very painful to sit. Normally uric acid is eliminated by the kidneys. If they are not functioning properly, the uric acid builds up.

Treatment A change in diet can help to reduce the pain and swelling. The Spleen-Pancreas meridian of the big toe is often the source of the problem. Work on the Through-going Vessel and the Yin Linking Vessel, then stimulate the Spleen-Pancreas Source Point (*Taihaku*). If this point is swollen and painful, simply place your hand on it.

GALLSTONES

Like diabetes and gout, gall stones result from a high-calorie diet containing too much animal fat and sugar. Symptoms appear on the right side of the diaphragm and along the right shoulder blade. According to the Yellow Emperor, the Gall Bladder functions like a judge, making decisions and handing down sentences. People who develop gall stones often make serious decisions, deal with considerable stress, and wine and dine luxuriously.

Treatment The Gall Bladder and the Liver are coupled in oriental medicine and exert a profound influence on one another. So work on the Belt Vessel and the Yang Linking Vessel meridians that connect them. People with gall stones suffer acute periodic pain, but it does not exhaust them as does hepatitis. Advise them to do meridian stretching exercises when the pain has ebbed.

HERNIA

The hernia of an intervertebral disc is, like whiplash, a common problem, especially among office workers and those who spend considerable time at their desks. It is also common among people who lift heavy objects, straining the lumbar or cervical spine. People with disc problems often live particularly stressful lives, eat strong rich food at irregular times and take little exercise.

Treatment Work on the Gall Bladder and Belt Vessel meridians, especially the leg circulation points. Work on the Bladder meridian on the back is also beneficial, but be sure to press extremely gently if there is any pain. In cases of extreme pain, leave this area alone, for fear of an adverse reaction. To re-establish good health, it is important to stabilize the patient's eating habits, stretch the meridians, exercise and have regular Shiatsu treatments.

HEPATITIS A AND B

These are Liver disorders caused by two different forms of an infectious virus. Symptoms include tiredness, loss of appetite, fever and the feeling of having caught a cold and, in some cases, jaundice. These symptoms normally disappear in six to eight weeks. Chronic hepatitis can be much more severe and more difficult to cure.

The Yellow Emperor portrayed the Liver as a general controlling an army. It defends the body against external aggression, replenishes the blood and renews the spirit (*kon*) that dwells within it. Modern medicine states that the liver stores and filters blood, converts and stores sugar and controls a range of delicate metabolic functions.

Treatment Serious liver problems demand medical attention. You can alleviate some of the symptoms and help the healing process by working on the Yin and Yang Linking Vessels. Work very gently when the patient is fatigued.

CHRONIC HEPATITIS

This condition is caused by either the A or B virus. The B virus in particular is said to become more virulent as it becomes chronic. It can lead to cirrhosis, so patients are advised to have a medical check-up.

Treatment This condition can be helped by regular Shiatsu treatments and meridian stretching exercises.

Patients should avoid alcohol, chocolate, sweets and any food with chemical additives.

HYPERTENSION

Hypertension (or high blood pressure) is linked with arteriosclerosis, a hardening and thickening of the smaller arteries. This causes the heart to pump harder. Higher blood pressure is the obvious result.

Blood pressure is a barometer of health. A recent Japanese survey comparing people's ages and diets showed that salty foods, excessive carbohydrates and alcohol weakened blood vessels and increased blood pressure, leading to a drop in life expectancy. As people grow older their blood pressure rises, usually because of clogging of the blood vessels that weaken and lose their elasticity. If they rupture, they can cause a brain haemorrhage or heart attack.

Treatment Shiatsu can help the blood circulate freely, regularize blood pressure and strengthen the blood vessels. Work on the Yin Linking Vessel for blood pressure problems, and on the Governing Vessel to help circulation. Very gentle pressure should be used in the treatment of an elderly person, particularly when they are on medication.

INFERTILITY

This is growing more and more common. Both physiological factors, such as obstruction of the Fallopian tubes or low sperm count, and psychological factors play a part in this problem. A recent Swedish survey showed a link between environment pollution, stress and the decline in the sperm count.

Treatment Shiatsu can diminish stress and restore potency. Work particularly with the Governing Vessel and the Conception Vessel and use the stretching exercises for both vessels. Ideally, a couple should do these exercises together and work on each other's meridians. A good Shiatsu therapist can help.

INSOMNIA

Such sleep problems afflict many who live in large cities or are under great stress. Though often people say that they do not sleep when they actually do, many are seriously affected by pathological insomnia and the terror of the 'white night'.

We cannot live more than five or six days without sleep. We begin to disintegrate, both psychologically and physically, and this well-known fact is often used in various forms of torture. Pathological sleeping disorders can be caused by trauma, a serious accident or a horrible experience. Light or superficial sleep usually results from too much 'head work', lack of exercise, irregular hours or environmental noise. If we do not have a regular sleeping pattern, it is easy to accumulate fatigue and fall into a serious illness. It is very important to build a regular sleeping pattern. *The Yellow Emperor's Classic of Internal Medicine* gives us a rationale for this, an analysis of energy flow in terms of the different hours of day and night.

According to the Yellow Emperor, from 4.00 until 12.00 is Large Yang; from 12.00 until 20.00 is Small Yin; from 0.00 until 02.00 is Large Yin; and from 2.00 until 4.00 is Small Yang. The most still and restorative part of the day (Large Yin) is between 0.00 and 2.00, when even trees and plants are sleeping. This is the most critical time to restore and renew your energy. Interestingly, this time is also connected with the Gall Bladder and the Liver meridians. The Liver is a great reservoir of the blood, restoring and filling it with dynamic energy. This restored blood then passes to the Lungs, associated with 3.00 to 5.00, another great energizer.

This shows that our most effective sleeping pattern should include the hours from about 22.00 until 4.00 or 5.00, the time when our energy can be most effectively recharged and restored. These are the hours of sleep in a traditional Zen monastery. We, of course, do not live in a monastery, but if we try to include the hours between 0.00 and 7.00 in our schedule of sleep, we will include the most deeply restorative times of the diurnal cycle.

Treatment People who have disturbed sleeping patterns, such as women who are recovering from childbirth, can do the Governing Vessel stretching exercise and work on the Heart Constrictor and the Heart meridians. Sleep, along with breathing, eating and elimination, is one of the vital physiological functions. Simply by changing our pattern of sleep, by sleeping better, we can significantly reduce many potentially dangerous hazards to our health.

LASSITUDE

You may feel languid and easily tired when you are faced with serious problems. They can also come from the autonomic nervous system or from psychological tension. Lack of appetite and general debility may indicate hepatitis or diabetes. According to oriental medicine, the feeling of tiredness is associated with the Liver function and is linked with the muscles, tendons and ligaments. Your toenails show the state of the Liver function, especially the toenail of the big toe where the Liver meridian lies.

Remember, organic problems build up slowly, accumulating until we are forced to pay attention to them. If the lassitude is severe, consult a doctor to identify which organs are involved.

Treatment The symptoms (restless sleep, irregular meals, stress, overstudy or overwork) can be treated by doing the Governing Vessel exercise fifty times each night before you go to sleep. Fortunately, this exercise does not require much physical effort. Use your body weight to swing yourself. Do this exercise in your bed if it is fairly hard; otherwise use a folded blanket on the floor.

MENOPAUSE

The menopause marks the cessation of the menstrual cycle. It normally occurs at age fifty, but this will vary depending on when puberty began. Menopause begins when the pituitary or master gland loses balanced contact with the ovaries. This affects the hypothalamus, which controls the autonomic nervous system, and can cause ataxia (lack of co-ordination between the sympathetic and parasympathetic nervous systems), palpitations, perspiration, dizziness, shoulder tension, vomiting and hot and cold flushes. When it affects the cerebral cortex, it produces mood swings, depression, apathy, irritation and forgetfulness. The Yellow Emperor describes two cycles, one for women and one for men, the woman's cycle beginning with puberty at age fourteen and ending with menopause at forty-nine.

Treatment Shiatsu treatment can help create a smooth transition from the menstrual cycle to menopause. Work on the Conception and Through-going Vessels, which correspond to puberty and menopause. The stretching exercises associated with these meridians will help considerably with the psychological problems associated with the change of life.

IRREGULAR MENSTRUATION

This is usually caused by hormonal imbalance or psychological tension. In oriental medicine, excessive menstruation is caused by excess energy (*jitsu*) and is often accompanied by heavy blood flow, intense abdominal pain, constipation and dizziness. Late menstruation is caused by lack of energy (*kyo*) and is accompanied by tiredness, scanty blood flow, mild pain and pale skin. Note that men need to take more exercise to compensate for the fact they have no monthly cycle to rid them of accumulating toxins.

Treatment The Spleen-Pancreas meridian and Spleen-Pancreas Point 6 (*Saninko*) can stimulate the cleansing process that takes place through the discharge of blood.

MISCARRIAGE

Miscarriages have three main causes: uterine contraction, haemorrhage and dilation of the cervix. When bleeding or pain occurs during pregnancy, medical attention is needed at once. Women who have had a miscarriage are often extremely apprehensive when they become pregnant again.

Treatment Shiatsu treatment can help these women. Work on the Through-going Vessel, the Conception Vessel and the Yin Linking Vessel. The Yin Linking Vessel in particular can help psychological tension. This Extraordinary Meridian is invaluable when treating someone who has already had a miscarriage.

MULTIPLE SCLEROSIS

This condition is a very serious central nervous system disorder. Symptoms include speech disturbances, impaired vision and muscular co-ordination, extreme fatigue and weakness. Some sufferers deteriorate quickly while others have relapses followed by periods of improvement. Shiatsu cannot cure this disorder, but it can slow the process of deterioration and provide psychological help to the patient. In advanced stages, someone who suffers from multiple sclerosis becomes completely discouraged, overwhelmed by feelings of weakness, helplessness and dependence.

Treatment These patients need a strong source of yang energy to help them. Work on the Governing Vessel and the Yang Ankle Vessel to promote and increase this circulation. The Yang Ankle Vessel is linked with the eyes, so work on the leg part of this meridian to bring energy into the eyes. Take particular care when working on Governing Vessel points on the vertebrae, because the patient may experience intense pain when pressure is applied here. Work gently, and avoid treating someone who is tired or shaking. Treatments should be no longer than thirty minutes. As with all serious problems, consult the patient's doctor for a clear diagnosis and decisions about treatment.

NEPHRITIS

This is an inflammation of the kidneys, accompanied by oedema, fever, pouches under the eyes, dark urine and high blood pressure. The urine contains both red and white blood cells. In oriental medicine, the kidneys are linked with other organs that, together, clean and distribute body fluids, and the Lung meridian controls evaporation of body fluids through the skin. When the Lung meridian and the kidneys are not functioning together properly, the arms and legs swell. The Spleen-Pancreas meridian produces large amounts of fluid. If it does not function properly, this fluid stagnates throughout the body, producing a characteristic swelling in the legs. The kidneys filter and flush fluid waste for the entire body. If they malfunction, the inner environment becomes poisonous. The two kidneys have slightly different functions. The right or yang kidney creates urine, while the left or yin kidney filters water.

Treatment To treat the kidneys, work on the Through-going Vessel, the Yin Ankle Vessel and the Conception Vessel. The Yin Linking Vessel is of great help in acute cases.

OBESITY

Obesity is linked with the excessive intake of fats and sugars coupled with a lack of exercise. It is particularly common in the industrialized nations. Though we do not die from obesity, it contributes directly to heart disease, circulatory problems and kidney failure. Fat also makes many people think they are ugly and complicates psychological problems.

The world is full of weight-loss clinics, which means there are a great number of people who have this problem. Shiatsu is a very effective way to reduce it, as I have seen time and again, though deep fat deposits can be tenacious. The miracles offered by those who use drugs to alter the metabolism are usually very short-lived. Our bodies have the natural capacity to reduce fat, just as they naturally accumulated it.

Treatment The patient's diet must be regulated, reducing fats and sugars, while the amount of exercise is increased. The Conception Vessel, Yang Ankle Vessel and Belt Vessel stretching exercises are all extremely effective.

PARKINSON'S DISEASE

This disease normally develops late in life, though, as with multiple sclerosis, younger people may be affected. Symptoms include muscle tremors and weakness, deterioration of the control of voluntary movements and copious sweating.

Treatment Since Parkinson's disease affects older people, the patient's muscles may have already become stiff and hard to work with. You can, however, put pressure on the Governing Vessel, Yang Ankle Vessel and Yang Linking Vessel points. Someone with Parkinson's disease will gradually stiffen into a foetal position. Work must be done to prevent this stiffening. Though working with the meridians may be difficult, with patience you can achieve quite a bit. Similarly, though the patient's speech may be jumbled and hard to understand, by listening carefully and working gently the practitioner can greatly slow the process of deterioration.

PYELITIS

This is a pelvic inflammation that occurs in the urethra. It is often caused by a bacterial infection, and is more frequent in women because a woman's shorter urethra is more vulnerable to infection. Symptoms include chills, high temperature and backache.

Treatment Avoid work on this condition when symptoms are acute. In severe cases, call a doctor. Work on the Through-going Vessel, Yin Ankle Vessel and Conception Vessel. As in kidney cases, the Yin Linking Vessel is extremely helpful in acute cases.

SCHIZOPHRENIA

This is a Greek word meaning *divided mind*. A schizophrenic may hallucinate, say ambivalent things, express overwhelming guilt or injure himself. It can be very frightening to watch. Because Shiatsu does not recognize this split between the mind and body, it can be of help in these problems.

Treatment Working on the Governing Vessel has a dramatic effect on mental problems. In oriental medicine, the unified personality is linked to the Heart meridian. Mental problems come from unintegrated parts of the personality, and working on the Governing Vessel's Regulating Point (the Small Intestine Point at the wrist) helps in this integration, for the Small Intestine is coupled with the Heart meridian. Mental problems are quite subtle, but one thing has become very clear to me through my own work: when the physical condition improves, the mind improves, though there may be no rational explanation.

STIFF SHOULDERS

The pain and discomfort associated with stiff shoulders are very common as we grow older. The Japanese call this *gojugata* or 'fiftieth shoulder', for many people find that their shoulders become stiff and painful around the age of fifty. The trapezius muscle tightens and the neck becomes so stiff it is hard to move your head or raise your arm, and vision can be impaired. Shiatsu can release tension in the muscles and restore freedom of movement.

Treatment Stiff shoulders in women can occur as a response to gynaecological problems. The reaction appears in the Small Intestine meridian, between the superior angle of the scapula and the first and second thoracic vertebrae. When the cause is systemic, the approach should be more global. Work on the Conception Vessel and the Through-going Vessel, both of which are directly linked to gynecological problems.

TONSILLITIS

The inflammation of the tonsils, organs that separate the passage between the nose and throat, can be so painful that it becomes impossible to eat and requires surgical intervention. Tonsillitis can be caused by an overabundance of rich food. It demands that the patient rest.

Treatment Work on the Large Intestine meridian, the Triple Warmer meridian and the Kidney meridian. You will normally feel a strong reaction on the Yang Linking Vessel meridian and the Yin Linking Vessel meridian. The source point (*gokoku*) of the Large Intestine meridian will be very sensitive. This inflammation is a vigorous effort on the part of the body to eliminate toxins.

ULCERS, DUODENAL

Duodenal ulcers are found where gastric juices attack the mucous membrane of the duodenum. The pain usually appears just after eating. If the pain is severe, be very careful about applying any pressure and patients are advised to consult a doctor.

Introverted people are particularly susceptible to ulcers, for they tend to swallow their problems. In oriental medicine, mind and body profoundly influence each other. The Stomach meridian (which includes the duodenum) is linked with the emotional and psychological features that reflect your inner thoughts, the thoughts that are held inside your heart.

Treatment Concentrate on the Stomach meridian, the second line of the Bladder meridian and the Yang Ankle Vessel.

ULCERS, STOMACH

Stomach ulcers are similar to duodenal ulcers but are found in the stomach. They are a common problem in Japan, where people eat fast, chew little and live under constant pressure. Japanese society is a hierarchy. Despite signs of change, tradition and conformity carry great weight. There is a tremendous pressure on the individual to conform to society's rules. It is this pressure that produces ulcers.

Treatment Work on the Stomach, Spleen-Pancreas and Yang Ankle Vessel meridians. Concentrate particularly on the Bladder meridian, both lines, from the third to the eleventh and twelfth thoracic vertebrae. Stomach Point 36 (*Sanri*) is very helpful. Patients should be *strenuously* told to avoid coffee, tea and white sugar, which contain strong irritants.

WHIPLASH

Whiplash resulting from a car accident can lead to nausea, double vision, severe headaches, neck pains and numbness in the arms, as well as buzzing in the ears that can last for years. It often occurs as a displacement between the fourth and fifth cervical vertebrae. The first four cervical vertebrae are much more fragile than the lower ones. They have great mobility and serve as a lash, while the lower three neck vertebrae serve as the fixed handle of the whip. Many meridians pass through the neck, so people suffering from whiplash often display symptoms on the Small Intestine, Triple Warmer and Gall Bladder meridians in the neck. Because whiplash is closely linked with the yang meridians, particularly the Triple Warmer and Gall Bladder meridians, it can cause headaches, double vision, and buzzing in the ears.

Treatment Work on the Governing Vessel, the Yang Ankle Vessel and the Yang Linking Vessel meridians. Accidents, like whiplash, can be more than just strange coincidences. They often contain a deep psychological content. Reflection can reveal their hidden causes. Patients should be encouraged to meditate on the accident. No one can predict an accident or a death, but in looking back you can often see where things went wrong and became unbalanced. Making this conscious can have a profound healing effect.

Glossary

Breathing is a very important way to control the flow of energy through the body. *Heaven* energy enters the body when inhaling. Exhaling expels poisons, breaks up preconceived ideas and rids you of out-moded habits.

Divination and diagnosis have much in common. In the east, diviners were thought to be wise and insightful people, and divination offered people images they could live by, symbols that connected them with the spirit. Doctors were thought to do just the same thing. They did not have to guess exactly which disease a person's symptoms indicated, but were more concerned with what these symptoms meant in the frame of the person's whole life. See *Sho*, *Shiyoho* and *Shinsen-jitsu*.

Earth is the ground we walk on and the power of *yin* in our bodies, the power to give things form. Earth can be very dangerous, for it is the cause of our death, the elimination of *yang*, yet today we are in danger of losing the Way or *Tao* of earth, for in its place we have deified our own intellect. Without earth there is no life. Without love of this planet we will soon die. We must recognize this and treasure the earth in its turn.

Essential Shiatsu is a perspective on *Shiatsu* that includes the wisdom of the *I Ching* and the radical practices associated with the *Eight Extraordinary Meridians*. It is based on the idea of freely circulating the energy of *heaven* and *earth* in your body. *Yo* means to nourish, *sei* is your physical life force, *do* is the Way. Essential Shiatsu means harmonizing your life energy by personally experiencing the interaction of heaven and earth.

Extraordinary Meridians The Eight Extraordinary Meridians are energy conduits that come to the rescue of the normal channels of our body (*Principal Meridians*) when they are overloaded. They can eliminate stress or provide much needed support to a system or an organ in danger. They are of particular importance in a time of stress like our own.

The **Five Processes** or **Five Elements** belong to an old Chinese system of analyzing process flow that was codified about 400 BCE. It has become crucial to oriental medicine. The five elements are organic processes that rotate in a sequence: fire, earth, metal, water and wood. They are associated with organs, seasons, directions, colours, tastes, diseases, political and emotional events. In *Shiatsu* they are used to show how the various circles of organs and organ meridians interact. The basic directions of the circle of processes are two: if you follow the circle around, you see a constructive evolution; if you cut across the middle of the circle to form the line of a star, you see a destructive process.

Governing points or source points are places where an entire *meridian* can be stimulated. They are particularly important as preparation for the stretching exercises associated with each of the *Extraordinary Meridians*.

Gua is the name of the diagrams of the *I Ching*. These begin with the opened and solid lines that indicate *yin* and *yang* and go on to include eight three-line figures or *trigrams* and the sixty-four six-line figures or *hexagrams*. Each of these *gua* symbolizes a moment of time. They are first of all used in divination, where they can answer a question you ask. They are also used in medicine and philosophy to talk about the way energy flows in *heaven* and *earth*.

Harmony is a great ideal of eastern thought and medicine. In *Shiatsu* it is expressed as the balance between *yin* and *yang*. Everything we do in working on the various *meridians* is aimed at restoring the primal balance between *heaven* and *earth*. Harmony is also philosophical. The healing process that restores the primal balance includes a way to think about yourself as something larger than your ego concerns. You must strive to see yourself as serving the *Tao*, or Way of Heaven.

Heaven is the world of spirit in eastern thought, giving us the gift of life and the ability to perceive things. Heaven is an ideal that can free us from the confines of our ego. It is light, inspiration and creative thought. The *Tao*, or Way of Heaven, is something that each person can experience every day in the movements of energy in their body. The Mandate of Heaven, an old Chinese idea, states that nothing can be accomplished in this world unless the power of heaven is with you.

Heaven and earth (*t'ien ti*) is the Chinese expression for the world we experience. It shows that all life is an interaction between spirit and form, and that the world we live in is continually being created. There is a wonderful image for this. Our world is like an enormous turtle swimming the warm seas of chaos. His upper shell is the overarching heavens, his lower shell (which the old Chinese used for divination) is the wide expanse of earth. We, the humans, are the soft flesh between them. We are a product of the connection of *heaven* (*t'ien*) and *earth* (*ti*).

A **hexagram** is a six-line diagram from the *I Ching* that describes a field of actions and associations. We can use the hexagrams and the trigrams of *I Ching* to understand how energy moves in the body.

I Ching (the *Book of Change* or the *Classic of Change*) is one of the oldest books in the world. It is a *divination* system that lets us know what we can do to live in accord with the *Tao* or Way. It is made up of sixty-four *gua* and their texts that portray archetypal shapes of time. Because it speaks in terms of *yin* and *yang* it also gives us a picture of how energy moves in the world. Many philosophers have seen the *I Ching* as an ideal way to live, a reflection of the *Tao* or Way of *Heaven*.

Ki is energy, the energy present in all things. Everything has *ki* or it could not exist. Thus everything is alive and interconnected. To become aware of *ki* is a very important step to both effective *Shiatsu* and general enlightenment. We think of *ki* as manifesting through *yin* and *yang*, and the energy that courses through the *meridians* and gives us life is *ki*. This energy can become imbalanced. It is the purpose of *Shiatsu* to help restore this balance.

A **meridian** is a path or conduit that conducts energy through the body. It connects with major organs and helps to control the flow of *yin* and *yang* energies throughout the system. Each meridian connects many pressure points where we can help to adjust energy flow. There are twelve *Principal Meridians* and eight *Extraordinary Meridians*. Each meridian has a *source point* or Governing Point through which it can be stimulated.

Principal Meridians are the basic channels through which energy flows in our body. They connect and interconnect organs and provide the conduits through which the various parts of our body communicate. The Principal Meridians can be easily overloaded and break down, thus creating an emergency situation in our body. At such time, the intervention of the *Extraordinary Meridians* becomes indispensible.

Shiatsu is a form of therapy that involves loving contact, manipulation of specific points on the body, and a series of stretches and exercises. Shiatsu manipulation uses the thumbs and the palms of the hands to put pressure on a particular *meridian* to adjust the balance of *yin* and *yang* within an individual and promote a free flow of *ki* energy.

Since the dawn of time there existed different ways of caring for the body in China. Shiatsu grew out of combining old Japanese healing methods such as *ankyo* and *do-in*, which stimulated energy flow in the meridians, with Chinese forms of acupuncture and herbal medicine. In the 1920s, it was recognized by the Japanese government as an official form of medicine.

Shiatsu is a way to live with the interconnections between *heaven* and *earth* as they are manifested in your own body. Today our relationship to heaven and earth is disharmonious. This imbalance is caused by human beings. If we are to live harmoniously with heaven and earth we must develop personal insight and an understanding of their delicate balance. If we can experience this intricate harmony, we may be able to find a way to successfully participate in it.

Shinsen-jitsu is a Japanese word meaning 'understanding the preservation of human vital force'. It lies behind all of our diagnostic practices. We must always remember that we are not attacking a specific disease but are trying to adjust a very important spiritual balance that has repercussions throughout a person's life.

Shiyoho is the contrary of *sho*. As an evaluation of diagnosis, it proposes a specific fit between observed symptoms and the elimination of those symptoms. Disease itself is the criterion, not what we call spiritual health.

Sho means the proof of a diagnosis. It suggests that the diagnosis has been of value to the sick person. It does not mean that the doctor has diagnosed a specific disease and made a specific cure. *Sho* is deeper, suggesting that the diagnosis and treatment is of spiritual value to the patient. This kind of work is our ideal.

Source point see *governing points*.

Tao is the most important idea in eastern philosophy. It means 'way' and suggests that the movement of the spirit, the Way of *Heaven*, offers an individual path or way for each person. A western thinker has called Tao the 'on-going process of the real'. Tao means that we try to live according to the Way of Heaven rather than our own ego, and it connects the overall 'way' of the world to the decisions we make every day. Through Tao those everyday moves can not only heal our own imbalances but contribute to the regeneration of the world around us.

Trigram is a three-line diagram from the *I Ching*. There are eight trigrams (*bagua*) that serve to connect a wide range of associations directly to our work with the body and its yin and yang balances.

The Yellow Emperor's Classic of Internal Medicine is a fundamental text in oriental medicine, compiled about the second century AD. It combines specific information on various styles of treatment, including a unique analysis of dreamwork, with a precise description of the *meridians* and a philosophical outlook that is shown to be as healing as the treatments.

Yang is active energy, spirit force, the energy of heaven, light, hot, dry, focused, driving, creative. Crucial for the preservation of life, yang is only imaginable in a pair with *yin*. It contains yin as a potential and, when it reaches its maximum, gives birth to yin. The *meridians* are organized in pairs of yin and yang. Yang meridians protect, yin meridians sustain from within. Health can be seen as a balance between yin and yang energies, just as sickness results from an imbalance in these two primal energies.

Yin is receptive energy, the energy of earth, shadowy dark, moist, cold, deathly. It gives birth to the *Five Processes:* wood, fire, earth, metal, water. Yin, when it reaches its maximum, gives birth to yang. Yin meridians sustain from within. Health can be seen as a balance between yin and yang energies, just as sickness results from their imbalance.